IBS-IBD Fiber Charts:

Soluble & Insoluble Fibre Data
for Over 450 Items,
Including Links to Internet Resources

By Kathy Steinemann

Print Edition
ISBN 978-1535152235

Foreword by D. Lee Jackson

Cover by Kathy Steinemann

Disclaimer

The material provided in this book is for informational purposes only. It is not meant to replace proper medical diagnosis, treatment, or advice. Always consult your physician and other appropriate health-care providers before taking any medications, natural remedies, or supplements; or before changing your diet. Discuss all plans, symptoms, and medical conditions with your doctor.

Any use of the ideas contained herein is at your own discretion, risk, and responsibility. The author assumes no liability for any of the information presented. There are no representations or warranties, either express or implied.

You should not begin or discontinue medical treatment based on information contained in this, or any other, book.

Also by this Author:

The IBS Compass: Contains all the fiber data and information from this book, plus numerous tips for coping with IBS, a link to a free self-hypnosis script, and a selection of recipes developed by the author.

Table of Contents

Foreword

By D. Lee Jackson

If you are reading this, you most likely know that irritable bowel syndrome makes life difficult. Aside from the obvious physical effects, it can play havoc with your mental health.

Nothing is more depressing than missing out on your favorite activities just because your guts are in turmoil.

I have lived with IBS-D since my eighth-grade days back in 1976. Over time, doctors have given me various less-than-helpful recommendations for how to control the symptoms. The most infuriating suggestion was when doctors (note the plural here) refused to acknowledge it as a physical ailment, saying I simply had "too much stress" in my life.

You bet I had too much stress. Can you guess what was causing it? Hint: It rhymes with *mama mia,* a word you might exclaim during a particularly bad attack.

Kathy Steinemann's *IBS-IBD Fiber Charts* was born from her own experience with IBS. She found that soluble fiber helped her condition, but simultaneously learned that information on the amounts of soluble fiber in foods was next to impossible to find. Her subsequent research has resulted in a book containing the percentages of soluble and insoluble fiber in more than 450 foods, both raw and commercially processed. It is a book I wish had been available when I was in college, when I could finally control my own diet. I have a feeling my life from that point onward might have been much easier.

—D. Lee Jackson

D. Lee Jackson is a Texas native, born in Austin in 1963. His wife and son have both had to learn to deal with his IBS-D symptoms. He is best known for his work on videogame soundtracks, having written music for *Rise of the Triad* and *Duke Nukem 3D*, including the latter's famous theme song, "Grabbag". He is now on disability retirement and is using the time to write his first novel.

Be sure to read his tongue-in-cheek advice, "How not to Prepare for a Colonoscopy", on page 55.

You can see his Wikipedia entry at:

https://en.wikipedia.org/wiki/Lee_Jackson_(composer)

Why I Wrote This Book

By Kathy Steinemann

I am not a doctor, naturopath, faith healer, acupuncturist, or health-food fanatic.

I'm someone just like you, someone whose life has been turned upside down by IBS.

Before I was formally diagnosed, I received little help from my medical doctor other than being told to avoid *roughage*. I had no idea of what roughage is, so I investigated.

Roughage is insoluble fiber, often scratchy in texture.

Many dozens of hours spent online and reading books about IBS made me realize that not all fiber is created equal. I needed to increase my intake of soluble fiber, the soothing substance that turns into a gel and helps to calm an irritated digestive system.

It was impossible to find a book with complete fiber data.

Spreadsheet to the rescue.

I compiled data from multiple sources, including food labels, government publications, and manufacturers' websites. At times, I e-mailed manufacturers directly. If I found multiple entries for a single food item, I analyzed the value ranges and discarded anything that looked excessively high or low when compared with the list. At that point, I ended up with several mid-range entries and picked one based on common sense and previous research.

The result of my efforts is this book. I hope it will help everyone who is interested in monitoring fiber intake. Take a copy with you wherever you go.

Make some informed decisions and get on with living!

PS: Did you notice that the title contains the words *fiber* and *fibre*? It was done purposely to allow internet searches based on both US- and UK-English spellings.

How Much Fiber Do You Need?

I thought my diet included sufficient fiber, until I started to keep a food diary.

I was wrong.

Here are the recommended daily guidelines, as suggested by the IOM (Institute of Medicine of the National Academies).

Males

- 9-13 years—31 grams
- 14-50 years—38 grams
- 50+ years—30 grams

Females

- 9-18 years—26 grams
- 19-50 years—25 grams
- 50+ years—21 grams

Remember that as you increase fiber, you'll need to ingest enough liquids and water. If you don't, the fiber won't digest properly, and constipation may develop.

The IOM also presents information on recommended consumption of water, which includes all beverages as well as moisture in foods. However, their advice is to let thirst be your guide, with a general recommendation that women consume about 2.7 liters (91 ounces) and men about 3.7 liters (125 ounces) of water daily from all sources.

If you have watery diarrhea or are sweating due to hot weather or prolonged physical activity, you should increase fluid consumption. Be careful, however, as too much fluid can also cause problems.

How to Use the Charts

Abbreviations:

C—cup
ea—each
g—gram
in—inch
ins f—insoluble fiber
med—medium
oz—ounce
RTE—ready-to-eat
sol f—fiber
Supp—supplement
Tbsp—tablespoon
tsp—teaspoon
w/—with
w/o—without
WW—whole wheat

Here is an example of how each item is broken down in the fiber charts:

Food Item, 1/2 C
32% sol F, 4.7 g sol F, 10.1 g ins F, 14.8 tot g F, 68% ins F

Note that each food is identified in bold type on the first line, followed by the serving size.

The next line indicates the percentage of soluble fiber, followed by the amount in grams. Insoluble fiber is listed next, with total grams of fiber as the last entry.

If there is just a trace of soluble fiber in a specific food item, it is identified as *Trace of sol f,* with no breakdown of percentage or grams.

The percentage is the important figure.

No matter what the quantity of a food item, if you know the percentage of soluble fiber, you can calculate the grams by multiplying [percentage] x [total quantity].

Grains, Breads, Rice, Pasta

Amaranth, dry, 1/2 C
32% sol F, 4.7 g sol F, 10.1 g ins F, 14.8 tot g F, 68% ins F

Barley, cooked, 1/2 C
25% sol F, 1.0 g sol F, 3.0 g ins F, 4.0 tot g F, 75% ins F

Barley, dry, 1/2 C
22% sol F, 3.4 g sol F, 12.2 g ins F, 15.6 tot g F, 78% ins F

Biscuits, baking powder, buttermilk, 1 med
60% sol F, 0.3 g sol F, 0.2 g ins F, 0.5 tot g F, 40% ins F

Bran, corn, dry, 1/2 C
3% sol F, 0.8 g sol F, 30.8 g ins F, 31.6 tot g F, 97% ins F

Bran, oat, dry, 100 g
33% sol F, 5.0 g sol F, 10.0 g ins F, 15.0 tot g F, 67% ins F

Bran, rice, dry, 1/2 C
13% sol F, 1.6 g sol F, 10.8 g ins F, 12.4 tot g F, 87% ins F

Bran, wheat, dry, 1/4 C
Trace of sol F, 6.0 g ins F, 6.0 tot g F, 100% ins F

Bread, bagels, oat bran, 4 in
33% sol F, 0.7 g sol F, 1.3 g ins F, 2.0 tot g F, 67% ins F

Bread, bagels, white, 1 ea
38% sol F, 0.6 g sol F, 1.0 g ins F, 1.6 tot g F, 63% ins F

Bread, bagels, WW, 1 ea
29% sol F, 0.9 g sol F, 2.2 g ins F, 3.1 tot g F, 71% ins F

Bread, Boston brown, 1 slice
24% sol F, 0.5 g sol F, 1.6 g ins F, 2.1 tot g F, 76% ins F

Bread, bran, 1 slice
13% sol F, 0.2 g sol F, 1.3 g ins F, 1.5 tot g F, 87% ins F

Bread, buns, brown, 1 med
27% sol F, 0.4 g sol F, 1.1 g ins F, 1.5 tot g F, 73% ins F

Bread, buns, cracked wheat, 1 med
27% sol F, 0.4 g sol F, 1.1 g ins F, 1.5 tot g F, 73% ins F

Bread, buns, crescent (refrig dough), 1 ea
60% sol F, 0.3 g sol F, 0.2 g ins F, 0.5 tot g F, 40% ins F

Bread, buns, French, 1 med
58% sol F, 0.7 g sol F, 0.5 g ins F, 1.2 tot g F, 42% ins F

Bread, buns, hamburger, brown, 1 med
28% sol F, 0.5 g sol F, 1.3 g ins F, 1.8 tot g F, 72% ins F

Bread, buns, hamburger, white, 1 med
33% sol F, 0.4 g sol F, 0.8 g ins F, 1.2 tot g F, 67% ins F

Bread, buns, hamburger, WW, 1 med
11% sol F, 0.3 g sol F, 2.5 g ins F, 2.8 tot g F, 89% ins F

Bread, buns, hard, 1 med
33% sol F, 0.4 g sol F, 0.8 g ins F, 1.2 tot g F, 67% ins F

Bread, buns, hoagie, 1 med
29% sol F, 0.8 g sol F, 2.0 g ins F, 2.8 tot g F, 71% ins F

Bread, buns, hot dog, white, 1 ea
33% sol F, 0.4 g sol F, 0.8 g ins F, 1.2 tot g F, 67% ins F

Bread, buns, kaiser, 1 med
33% sol F, 0.4 g sol F, 0.8 g ins F, 1.2 tot g F, 67% ins F

Bread, buns, multigrain, 1 med
27% sol F, 0.4 g sol F, 1.1 g ins F, 1.5 tot g F, 73% ins F

Bread, buns, oat bran, 1 med
53% sol F, 0.8 g sol F, 0.7 g ins F, 1.5 tot g F, 47% ins F

Bread, buns, oatmeal, 1 med
55% sol F, 0.6 g sol F, 0.5 g ins F, 1.1 tot g F, 45% ins F

Bread, buns, pumpernickel, 1 med
52% sol F, 1.1 g sol F, 1.0 g ins F, 2.1 tot g F, 48% ins F

Bread, buns, rye, 1 med
52% sol F, 1.1 g sol F, 1.0 g ins F, 2.1 tot g F, 48% ins F

Bread, buns, sourdough, 1 med
67% sol F, 0.8 g sol F, 0.4 g ins F, 1.2 tot g F, 33% ins F

Bread, buns, Vienna, 1 med
58% sol F, 0.7 g sol F, 0.5 g ins F, 1.2 tot g F, 42% ins F

Bread, buns, white, 1 med
36% sol F, 0.4 g sol F, 0.7 g ins F, 1.1 tot g F, 64% ins F

Bread, buns, WW, 1 med
16% sol F, 0.4 g sol F, 2.1 g ins F, 2.5 tot g F, 84% ins F

Bread, cheese, 1 slice
60% sol F, 0.3 g sol F, 0.2 g ins F, 0.5 tot g F, 40% ins F

Bread, cinnamon swirl, 1 slice
50% sol F, 0.3 g sol F, 0.3 g ins F, 0.6 tot g F, 50% ins F

Bread, cornbread, 2-in cube
21% sol F, 0.3 g sol F, 1.1 g ins F, 1.4 tot g F, 79% ins F

Bread, cracked wheat, 1 slice
30% sol F, 0.3 g sol F, 0.7 g ins F, 1.0 tot g F, 70% ins F

Bread, dinner rolls, white, 1 roll
38% sol F, 0.3 g sol F, 0.5 g ins F, 0.8 tot g F, 63% ins F

Bread, egg, 1 slice
50% sol F, 0.2 g sol F, 0.2 g ins F, 0.4 tot g F, 50% ins F

Bread, flat, corn tortillas, 1 ea
29% sol F, 0.4 g sol F, 1.0 g ins F, 1.4 tot g F, 71% ins F

Bread, flat, tortillas, 6 in
15% sol F, 0.2 g sol F, 1.1 g ins F, 1.3 tot g F, 85% ins F

Bread, flour tortillas (wheat), RTE, 100 g
39% sol F, 0.9 g sol F, 1.4 g ins F, 2.4 tot g F, 61% ins F

Bread, focaccia, 1 slice
58% sol F, 0.7 g sol F, 0.5 g ins F, 1.2 tot g F, 42% ins F

Bread, French, 1 slice
40% sol F, 0.4 g sol F, 0.6 g ins F, 1.0 tot g F, 60% ins F

Bread, Hovis, 1 slice
33% sol F, 0.2 g sol F, 0.4 g ins F, 0.6 tot g F, 67% ins F

Bread, Italian, 1 slice
60% sol F, 0.3 g sol F, 0.2 g ins F, 0.5 tot g F, 40% ins F

Bread, matzo/matzah, 1 piece
50% sol F, 0.4 g sol F, 0.4 g ins F, 0.8 tot g F, 50% ins F

Bread, matzo/matzah, egg, 1 piece
63% sol F, 0.5 g sol F, 0.3 g ins F, 0.8 tot g F, 38% ins F

Bread, matzo/matzah, WW, 1 piece
50% sol F, 0.4 g sol F, 0.4 g ins F, 0.8 tot g F, 50% ins F

Bread, multigrain or granola, 1 slice
Trace of sol F, 2.0 g ins F, 2.0 tot g F, 100% ins F

Bread, oat bran, 1 slice
36% sol F, 0.4 g sol F, 0.7 g ins F, 1.1 tot g F, 64% ins F

Bread, oatmeal, 1 slice
25% sol F, 0.6 g sol F, 1.8 g ins F, 2.4 tot g F, 75% ins F

Bread, pita, white, 7 in
54% sol F, 0.7 g sol F, 0.6 g ins F, 1.3 tot g F, 46% ins F

Bread, pita, WW, 7 in
16% sol F, 0.7 g sol F, 3.7 g ins F, 4.4 tot g F, 84% ins F

Bread, pumpernickel, 1 slice
50% sol F, 0.5 g sol F, 0.5 g ins F, 1.0 tot g F, 50% ins F

Bread, raisin, 1 slice
25% sol F, 0.3 g sol F, 0.9 g ins F, 1.2 tot g F, 75% ins F

Bread, rye, 1 slice
44% sol F, 0.8 g sol F, 1.0 g ins F, 1.8 tot g F, 56% ins F

Bread, sourdough, 1 slice
32% sol F, 0.9 g sol F, 1.9 g ins F, 2.8 tot g F, 68% ins F

Bread, white, 1 slice
40% sol F, 0.2 g sol F, 0.3 g ins F, 0.5 tot g F, 60% ins F

Bread, WW, 1 slice
23% sol F, 0.5 g sol F, 1.7 g ins F, 2.2 tot g F, 77% ins F

Buckwheat groats, dry, 1/2 C
14% sol F, 1.2 g sol F, 7.3 g ins F, 8.5 tot g F, 86% ins F

Bulgur, cooked, 1/2 C
25% sol F, 1.0 g sol F, 3.0 g ins F, 4.0 tot g F, 75% ins F

Bulgur, dry, 1/2 C
17% sol F, 2.2 g sol F, 10.7 g ins F, 12.8 tot g F, 83% ins F

Crackers, graham, 2 ea
Trace of sol F, 1.4 g ins F, 1.4 tot g F, 100% ins F

Crackers, melba, 5 crackers
22% sol F, 0.4 g sol F, 1.4 g ins F, 1.8 tot g F, 78% ins F

Crackers, Ritz, 6 crackers
40% sol F, 0.2 g sol F, 0.3 g ins F, 0.5 tot g F, 60% ins F

Crackers, saltine, 1 oz
33% sol F, 0.4 g sol F, 0.8 g ins F, 1.2 tot g F, 67% ins F

Crackers, Triscuits, 1 oz
40% sol F, 0.2 g sol F, 0.3 g ins F, 0.5 tot g F, 60% ins F

Crackers, Wheat Thins, 1 oz
25% sol F, 0.3 g sol F, 0.9 g ins F, 1.2 tot g F, 75% ins F

Flour, arrowroot, 1/2 C
2% sol F, 0.1 g sol F, 2.1 g ins F, 2.2 tot g F, 98% ins F

Flour, barley, 1/2 C
22% sol F, 1.7 g sol F, 5.9 g ins F, 7.5 tot g F, 78% ins F

Flour, barley bran, 1/2 C
4% sol F, 2.2 g sol F, 47.9 g ins F, 50.0 tot g F, 96% ins F

Flour, barley malt, 1/2 C
22% sol F, 1.3 g sol F, 4.5 g ins F, 5.8 tot g F, 78% ins F

Flour, buckwheat, 1/2 C
14% sol F, 0.9 g sol F, 5.2 g ins F, 6.0 tot g F, 86% ins F

Flour, cake or pastry, 1/2 C
52% sol F, 0.6 g sol F, 0.6 g ins F, 1.2 tot g F, 48% ins F

Flour, chickpea, 1/2 C
21% sol F, 1.1 g sol F, 3.9 g ins F, 5.0 tot g F, 79% ins F

Flour, corn, 1/2 C
44% sol F, 2.4 g sol F, 3.1 g ins F, 5.5 tot g F, 56% ins F

Flour, cornmeal, degermed, 100 g
16% sol F, 0.6 g sol F, 3.3 g ins F, 3.9 tot g F, 84% ins F

Flour, cornstarch, 100 g
93% sol F, 1.0 g sol F, 0.1 g ins F, 1.1 tot g F, 7% ins F

Flour, konjac, 1 tsp
100% sol F, 5.0 g sol F, 0.0 g ins F, 5.0 tot g F, 0% ins F

Flour, oat, 2.5 Tbsp
56% sol F, 1.0 g sol F, 0.8 g ins F, 1.8 tot g F, 44% ins F

Flour, peanut, low fat, 1/2 C
27% sol F, 1.3 g sol F, 3.5 g ins F, 4.8 tot g F, 73% ins F

Flour, potato, 1/2 C
54% sol F, 2.6 g sol F, 2.2 g ins F, 4.7 tot g F, 46% ins F

Flour, quinoa, 1/2 C
36% sol F, 2.2 g sol F, 3.8 g ins F, 6.0 tot g F, 64% ins F

Flour, rice, brown, 1/2 C
15% sol F, 0.6 g sol F, 3.1 g ins F, 3.7 tot g F, 85% ins F

Flour, rice, white, 1/2 C
33% sol F, 0.6 g sol F, 1.3 g ins F, 1.9 tot g F, 67% ins F

Flour, rye, 1/2 C
27% sol F, 2.0 g sol F, 5.5 g ins F, 7.5 tot g F, 73% ins F

Flour, soy, 1/2 C
44% sol F, 1.8 g sol F, 2.3 g ins F, 4.1 tot g F, 56% ins F

Flour, soy, defatted, 1/2 C
45% sol F, 4.0 g sol F, 4.8 g ins F, 8.8 tot g F, 55% ins F

Flour, teff, 1/2 C
Trace of sol F, 7.5 g ins F, 7.5 tot g F, 100% ins F

Flour, triticale, whole grain, 1/2 C
18% sol F, 1.8 g sol F, 7.8 g ins F, 9.5 tot g F, 82% ins F

Flour, white, 2.5 Tbsp
50% sol F, 0.3 g sol F, 0.3 g ins F, 0.6 tot g F, 50% ins F

Flour, white, all purp, bleached, 100 g
51% sol F, 1.5 g sol F, 1.5 g ins F, 3.0 tot g F, 49% ins F

Flour, WW, 2.5 Tbsp
14% sol F, 0.3 g sol F, 1.8 g ins F, 2.1 tot g F, 86% ins F

Muffins, blueberry, 1 med
44% sol F, 0.4 g sol F, 0.5 g ins F, 0.9 tot g F, 56% ins F

Muffins, bran, 1 med
12% sol F, 0.3 g sol F, 2.3 g ins F, 2.6 tot g F, 88% ins F

Muffins, carrot, 1 med
50% sol F, 0.5 g sol F, 0.5 g ins F, 1.0 tot g F, 50% ins F

Muffins, corn, 1 med
17% sol F, 0.2 g sol F, 1.0 g ins F, 1.2 tot g F, 83% ins F

Muffins, English, white, 1 ea
27% sol F, 0.4 g sol F, 1.1 g ins F, 1.5 tot g F, 73% ins F

Muffins, English, WW, 1 ea
18% sol F, 0.8 g sol F, 3.6 g ins F, 4.4 tot g F, 82% ins F

Muffins, oat bran or oatmeal, 1 med
50% sol F, 0.6 g sol F, 0.6 g ins F, 1.2 tot g F, 50% ins F

Pancakes, 1 med
11% sol F, 0.2 g sol F, 1.6 g ins F, 1.8 tot g F, 89% ins F

Pasta, egg noodles, cooked, 1/2 C
38% sol F, 0.3 g sol F, 0.5 g ins F, 0.8 tot g F, 63% ins F

Pasta, No Yolks, cooked, 1 1/2 C
10% sol F, 0.3 g sol F, 2.7 g ins F, 3.0 tot g F, 90% ins F

Pasta, rice noodles, cooked, 1/2 C
22% sol F, 0.2 g sol F, 0.7 g ins F, 0.9 tot g F, 78% ins F

Pasta, spaghetti, cooked, 1/2 C
Trace of sol F, 0.8 g ins F, 0.8 tot g F, 100% ins F

Pasta, spaghetti, WW, cooked, 1/2 C
25% sol F, 0.5 g sol F, 1.5 g ins F, 2.0 tot g F, 75% ins F

Pasta, spiral, cooked, 1/2 C
15% sol F, 0.1 g sol F, 0.6 g ins F, 0.7 tot g F, 85% ins F

Pasta, spiral, WW, cooked, 1/2 C
19% sol F, 0.4 g sol F, 1.5 g ins F, 1.9 tot g F, 81% ins F

Popcorn, popped, 3 C
29% sol F, 0.8 g sol F, 2.0 g ins F, 2.8 tot g F, 71% ins F

Psyllium husk, 10 g
89% sol F, 7.1 g sol F, 0.9 g ins F, 8.0 tot g F, 11% ins F

Quinoa, cooked, 1/2 C
13% sol F, 0.6 g sol F, 4.1 g ins F, 4.7 tot g F, 87% ins F

Quinoa, dry, 1/2 C
14% sol F, 0.7 g sol F, 4.0 g ins F, 4.7 tot g F, 86% ins F

Rice, brown, cooked, 1/2 C
11% sol F, 0.2 g sol F, 1.6 g ins F, 1.8 tot g F, 89% ins F

Rice, white, cooked, 1/2 C
33% sol F, 0.2 g sol F, 0.4 g ins F, 0.6 tot g F, 67% ins F

Rice, white, instant, cooked, 1/2 C
29% sol F, 0.1 g sol F, 0.3 g ins F, 0.4 tot g F, 71% ins F

Rice, wild, cooked, 1/2 C
15% sol F, 0.2 g sol F, 1.1 g ins F, 1.3 tot g F, 85% ins F

Scones, 1 med
43% sol F, 0.3 g sol F, 0.4 g ins F, 0.7 tot g F, 57% ins F

Sorghum, 1/2 C
30% sol F, 4.0 g sol F, 9.3 g ins F, 13.3 tot g F, 70% ins F

Wafers, rye, 3 ea
3% sol F, 0.1 g sol F, 2.2 g ins F, 2.3 tot g F, 97% ins F

Waffles, round, 4-in diameter, 1 ea
43% sol F, 0.3 g sol F, 0.4 g ins F, 0.7 tot g F, 57% ins F

Wheat, gluten, 1/2 C
Trace of sol F, 6.2 g ins F, 6.2 tot g F, 100% ins F

Wheat, spelt, 1/2 C
12% sol F, 0.8 g sol F, 6.1 g ins F, 6.9 tot g F, 88% ins F

Wheat, sprouted, 1/2 C
17% sol F, 0.1 g sol F, 0.5 g ins F, 0.6 tot g F, 83% ins F

Breakfast Cereals

100% Bran, 1/2 C
8% sol F, 1.0 g sol F, 11.0 g ins F, 12.0 tot g F, 92% ins F

All-Bran, 2/3 C
8% sol F, 1.0 g sol F, 12.0 g ins F, 13.0 tot g F, 92% ins F

All-Bran with Extra Fiber, 1/2 C
8% sol F, 1.0 g sol F, 12.0 g ins F, 13.0 tot g F, 92% ins F

Basic 4, 3/4 C
33% sol F, 1.0 g sol F, 2.0 g ins F, 3.0 tot g F, 67% ins F

Bran Buds, 1/3 C
25% sol F, 3.0 g sol F, 9.0 g ins F, 12.0 tot g F, 75% ins F

Bran Chex, Multi, 2/3 C
Trace of sol F, 4.0 g ins F, 4.0 tot g F, 100% ins F

Bran Flakes, without raisins, 3/4 C
Trace of sol F, 5.0 g ins F, 5.0 tot g F, 100% ins F

Bulger, cooked, 1/2 C
25% sol F, 1.0 g sol F, 3.0 g ins F, 4.0 tot g F, 75% ins F

Cheerios, 1/2 C
25% sol F, 0.3 g sol F, 0.8 g ins F, 1.0 tot g F, 75% ins F

Cheerios, Multigrain, 1/2 C
33% sol F, 0.5 g sol F, 1.0 g ins F, 1.5 tot g F, 67% ins F

Complete Bran Flakes, 3/4 C
Trace of sol F, 5.0 g ins F, 5.0 tot g F, 100% ins F

Complete Oat Bran Flakes, 2/3 C
33% sol F, 1.0 g sol F, 2.0 g ins F, 3.0 tot g F, 67% ins F

Corn Bran, 1/2 C
3% sol F, 0.1 g sol F, 3.8 g ins F, 4.0 tot g F, 97% ins F

Corn grits, cooked, 1/2 C
32% sol F, 0.6 g sol F, 1.3 g ins F, 1.9 tot g F, 68% ins F

Cornflakes, 1/2 C
Trace of sol F, 0.4 g ins F, 0.4 tot g F, 100% ins F

Cornmeal, cooked, 1/2 C
4% sol F, 0.1 g sol F, 1.3 g ins F, 1.4 tot g F, 96% ins F

Cornmeal, dry, 1/2 C
1% sol F, 0.1 g sol F, 5.1 g ins F, 5.1 tot g F, 99% ins F

Couscous, cooked, 1/2 C
22% sol F, 0.3 g sol F, 1.1 g ins F, 1.4 tot g F, 78% ins F

Couscous, dry, 1/2 C
22% sol F, 1.0 g sol F, 3.4 g ins F, 4.3 tot g F, 78% ins F

Cracked Wheat, cooked, 1/2 C
Trace of sol F, 3.0 g ins F, 3.0 tot g F, 100% ins F

Cracklin' Oat Bran, 1/3 C
Trace of sol F, 3.0 g ins F, 3.0 tot g F, 100% ins F

Cream of rice, cooked, 1/2 C
25% sol F, 0.1 g sol F, 0.2 g ins F, 0.2 tot g F, 75% ins F

Cream of Wheat, uncooked, 2.5 Tbsp
36% sol F, 0.4 g sol F, 0.7 g ins F, 1.1 tot g F, 64% ins F

Fiber One, 1/2 C
7% sol F, 1.0 g sol F, 13.0 g ins F, 14.0 tot g F, 93% ins F

Granola, low fat with raisins, 1/2 C
33% sol F, 1.0 g sol F, 2.0 g ins F, 3.0 tot g F, 67% ins F

Grape-Nuts Flakes, 3/4 C
Trace of sol F, 3.0 g ins F, 3.0 tot g F, 100% ins F

Heartland Granola, 1/4 C
50% sol F, 1.0 g sol F, 1.0 g ins F, 2.0 tot g F, 50% ins F

Just Right Fruit and Nut, 3/4 C
Trace of sol F, 2.0 g ins F, 2.0 tot g F, 100% ins F

Kasha, cooked, 1/2 C
13% sol F, 0.4 g sol F, 2.3 g ins F, 2.7 tot g F, 87% ins F

Kashi 7 Whole Grain Puffed Cereal , 1/2 C
Trace of sol F, 1.0 g ins F, 1.0 tot g F, 100% ins F

Kashi Heart to Heart, 3/4 C
20% sol F, 1.0 g sol F, 4.0 g ins F, 5.0 tot g F, 80% ins F

Millet, cooked, 1/2 C
18% sol F, 0.6 g sol F, 2.7 g ins F, 3.3 tot g F, 82% ins F

Millet, dry, 1/2 C
19% sol F, 1.6 g sol F, 6.9 g ins F, 8.5 tot g F, 81% ins F

Mueslix, 2/3 C
25% sol F, 1.0 g sol F, 3.0 g ins F, 4.0 tot g F, 75% ins F

Nature's Path Organic Corn Flakes, 3/4 C
Trace of sol F, 2.0 g ins F, 2.0 tot g F, 100% ins F

Nature's Path Organic Crispy Rice, 3/4 C
Trace of sol F, 2.0 g ins F, 2.0 tot g F, 100% ins F

Nutri-Grain-Golden Wheat, 3/4 C
Trace of sol F, 4.0 g ins F, 4.0 tot g F, 100% ins F

Oat bran, cooked, 3/4 C
55% sol F, 2.2 g sol F, 1.8 g ins F, 4.0 tot g F, 45% ins F

Oatmeal, cooked, 1/2 C
50% sol F, 1.0 g sol F, 1.0 g ins F, 2.0 tot g F, 50% ins F

Oatmeal, dry, 1/2 C
47% sol F, 2.0 g sol F, 2.3 g ins F, 4.3 tot g F, 53% ins F

Oatmeal, instant, cooked, 1/2 C
66% sol F, 0.8 g sol F, 0.4 g ins F, 1.3 tot g F, 34% ins F

Oats, rolled, cooked, 3/4 C
43% sol F, 1.3 g sol F, 1.7 g ins F, 3.0 tot g F, 57% ins F

Oats, whole, cooked, 1/2 C
31% sol F, 0.5 g sol F, 1.1 g ins F, 1.6 tot g F, 69% ins F

Original Frosted Mini-Wheats, 4 large
25% sol F, 1.0 g sol F, 3.0 g ins F, 4.0 tot g F, 75% ins F

Puffed Rice, 1/2 C
50% sol F, 0.3 g sol F, 0.3 g ins F, 0.5 tot g F, 50% ins F

Raisin Bran, 3/4 C
17% sol F, 1.0 g sol F, 5.0 g ins F, 6.0 tot g F, 83% ins F

Rice Krispies, 1/2 C
33% sol F, 0.1 g sol F, 0.1 g ins F, 0.2 tot g F, 67% ins F

Rolled wheat, cooked, 1/2 C
16% sol F, 0.3 g sol F, 1.3 g ins F, 1.6 tot g F, 84% ins F

Shredded Wheat, 2/3 C
14% sol F, 0.5 g sol F, 3.0 g ins F, 3.5 tot g F, 86% ins F

Smacks, 3/4 C
Trace of sol F, 1.0 g ins F, 1.0 tot g F, 100% ins F

Smart Start, 1/2 C
Trace of sol F, 1.0 g ins F, 1.0 tot g F, 100% ins F

Special K, 1/2 C
22% sol F, 0.1 g sol F, 0.4 g ins F, 0.5 tot g F, 78% ins F

Total, 1/2 C
25% sol F, 0.5 g sol F, 1.5 g ins F, 2.0 tot g F, 75% ins F

Total Raisin Bran, 1/2 C
15% sol F, 0.5 g sol F, 2.6 g ins F, 3.0 tot g F, 85% ins F

Wheat Chex, 2/3 C
20% sol F, 1.0 g sol F, 4.0 g ins F, 5.0 tot g F, 80% ins F

Wheat Germ, RTE, 1/4 C
25% sol F, 1.0 g sol F, 3.0 g ins F, 4.0 tot g F, 75% ins F

Wheaties, 1/2 C
50% sol F, 0.5 g sol F, 0.5 g ins F, 1.0 tot g F, 50% ins F

Vegetables, Legumes, Lentils

Artichokes, 1 globe
72% sol F, 4.7 g sol F, 1.8 g ins F, 6.5 tot g F, 28% ins F

Asparagus, cooked, 1/2 C
61% sol F, 1.7 g sol F, 1.1 g ins F, 2.8 tot g F, 39% ins F

Asparagus, raw, 1/2 C
39% sol F, 0.7 g sol F, 1.1 g ins F, 1.8 tot g F, 61% ins F

Sprouts, acorn, cooked, 1/2 C
57% sol F, 3.1 g sol F, 2.3 g ins F, 5.4 tot g F, 43% ins F

Sprouts, alfalfa, raw, 1/2 C
25% sol F, 0.1 g sol F, 0.2 g ins F, 0.3 tot g F, 75% ins F

Sprouts, bean, raw, 1/2 C
38% sol F, 0.3 g sol F, 0.5 g ins F, 0.8 tot g F, 63% ins F

Sprouts, mung bean, cooked, 1/2 C
60% sol F, 0.3 g sol F, 0.2 g ins F, 0.5 tot g F, 40% ins F

Sprouts, soybean, raw, 1/2 C
50% sol F, 0.2 g sol F, 0.2 g ins F, 0.4 tot g F, 50% ins F

Beans, baked, 1/2 C
50% sol F, 3.0 g sol F, 3.0 g ins F, 6.0 tot g F, 50% ins F

Beans, bayo, cooked, 1/2 C
40% sol F, 1.2 g sol F, 1.8 g ins F, 2.9 tot g F, 60% ins F

Beans, black, cooked, 1/2 C
39% sol F, 2.4 g sol F, 3.7 g ins F, 6.1 tot g F, 61% ins F

Beans, butter, cooked, 1/2 C
39% sol F, 2.7 g sol F, 4.2 g ins F, 6.9 tot g F, 61% ins F

Beans, chick beans, cooked, 1/2 C
21% sol F, 1.3 g sol F, 4.9 g ins F, 6.2 tot g F, 79% ins F

Beans, garbanzo, cooked, 1/2 C
21% sol F, 1.3 g sol F, 4.9 g ins F, 6.2 tot g F, 79% ins F

Beans, green, canned, 1/2 C
25% sol F, 0.5 g sol F, 1.5 g ins F, 2.0 tot g F, 75% ins F

Beans, green, cooked, 1/2 C
40% sol F, 0.8 g sol F, 1.2 g ins F, 2.0 tot g F, 60% ins F

Beans, green/string canned, 1/2 C
38% sol F, 0.5 g sol F, 0.8 g ins F, 1.3 tot g F, 62% ins F

Beans, kidney, cooked, 1/2 C
11% sol F, 0.5 g sol F, 4.0 g ins F, 4.5 tot g F, 89% ins F

Beans, lima, cooked, 1/2 C
43% sol F, 3.0 g sol F, 4.0 g ins F, 7.0 tot g F, 57% ins F

Beans, navy, cooked, 1/2 C
33% sol F, 2.0 g sol F, 4.0 g ins F, 6.0 tot g F, 67% ins F

Beans, northern, cooked, 1/2 C
25% sol F, 1.4 g sol F, 4.2 g ins F, 5.6 tot g F, 75% ins F

Beans, pinto, cooked, 1/2 C
26% sol F, 1.9 g sol F, 5.5 g ins F, 7.4 tot g F, 74% ins F

Beans, soy, cooked, 1/2 C
45% sol F, 2.3 g sol F, 2.8 g ins F, 5.1 tot g F, 55% ins F

Beans, string, cooked, 1/2 C
50% sol F, 1.0 g sol F, 1.0 g ins F, 2.0 tot g F, 50% ins F

Beans, white, cooked, 1/2 C
10% sol F, 0.4 g sol F, 3.8 g ins F, 4.2 tot g F, 90% ins F

Beet greens, cooked, 1/2 C
45% sol F, 1.0 g sol F, 1.2 g ins F, 2.1 tot g F, 55% ins F

Beet greens, raw, 1/2 C
29% sol F, 0.2 g sol F, 0.5 g ins F, 0.7 tot g F, 71% ins F

Beets, cooked, w/o skin, 1/2 C
46% sol F, 0.8 g sol F, 1.0 g ins F, 1.8 tot g F, 54% ins F

Beets, raw, w/o skin, 1/2 C
44% sol F, 0.8 g sol F, 1.0 g ins F, 1.8 tot g F, 56% ins F

Bok choy/pak choi, cooked, 1/2 C
37% sol F, 0.5 g sol F, 0.9 g ins F, 1.4 tot g F, 63% ins F

Bok choy/pak choi, raw, 1/2 C
43% sol F, 0.2 g sol F, 0.2 g ins F, 0.4 tot g F, 57% ins F

Broccoflower, cooked, 1/2 C
44% sol F, 0.6 g sol F, 0.8 g ins F, 1.4 tot g F, 56% ins F

Broccoflower, raw, 1/2 C
50% sol F, 0.5 g sol F, 0.5 g ins F, 1.0 tot g F, 50% ins F

Broccoli, cooked, 1/2 C
50% sol F, 1.2 g sol F, 1.2 g ins F, 2.4 tot g F, 50% ins F

Broccoli, raw, 100 g
13% sol F, 0.4 g sol F, 3.1 g ins F, 3.5 tot g F, 87% ins F

Brussels sprouts, cooked, 1/2 C
67% sol F, 2.0 g sol F, 1.0 g ins F, 3.0 tot g F, 33% ins F

Cabbage, green, cooked, 1/2 C
44% sol F, 0.8 g sol F, 1.0 g ins F, 1.7 tot g F, 56% ins F

Cabbage, green, raw, 1/2 C
44% sol F, 0.8 g sol F, 1.0 g ins F, 1.8 tot g F, 56% ins F

Cabbage, red, cooked, 1/2 C
43% sol F, 0.7 g sol F, 0.9 g ins F, 1.5 tot g F, 57% ins F

Cabbage, red, raw, 1/2 C
44% sol F, 0.4 g sol F, 0.5 g ins F, 0.9 tot g F, 56% ins F

Carrot juice, 1/2 C
26% sol F, 0.3 g sol F, 0.7 g ins F, 1.0 tot g F, 74% ins F

Carrots, canned, 1/2 C
47% sol F, 0.7 g sol F, 0.8 g ins F, 1.5 tot g F, 53% ins F

Carrots, cooked, 1/2 C
50% sol F, 1.0 g sol F, 1.0 g ins F, 2.0 tot g F, 50% ins F

Carrots, raw, 7.5 in
48% sol F, 1.1 g sol F, 1.2 g ins F, 2.3 tot g F, 52% ins F

Cassava (yuca), cooked, 1/2 C
40% sol F, 0.3 g sol F, 0.5 g ins F, 0.8 tot g F, 60% ins F

Cauliflower, cooked, 1/2 C
30% sol F, 0.6 g sol F, 1.4 g ins F, 2.0 tot g F, 70% ins F

Cauliflower, raw, 1/2 C
36% sol F, 0.5 g sol F, 0.8 g ins F, 1.3 tot g F, 64% ins F

Celeriac root, cooked, 1/2 C
47% sol F, 0.5 g sol F, 0.5 g ins F, 1.0 tot g F, 53% ins F

Celery, raw, chopped, 1/2 C
22% sol F, 0.2 g sol F, 0.7 g ins F, 0.9 tot g F, 78% ins F

Chard, cooked, 1/2 C
16% sol F, 0.3 g sol F, 1.6 g ins F, 1.9 tot g F, 84% ins F

Collard greens, cooked, 1/2 C
60% sol F, 1.6 g sol F, 1.1 g ins F, 2.7 tot g F, 40% ins F

Collard greens, raw, 1/2 C
62% sol F, 0.4 g sol F, 0.3 g ins F, 0.7 tot g F, 38% ins F

Corn, cooked, 1/2 C
13% sol F, 0.3 g sol F, 1.7 g ins F, 2.0 tot g F, 87% ins F

Corn, whole kernel, canned, 1/2 C
13% sol F, 0.2 g sol F, 1.4 g ins F, 1.6 tot g F, 88% ins F

Cucumbers, 1/2 C
25% sol F, 0.1 g sol F, 0.3 g ins F, 0.4 tot g F, 75% ins F

Eggplants, 1/2 C
25% sol F, 0.3 g sol F, 0.9 g ins F, 1.2 tot g F, 75% ins F

Fennel bulb, raw, 1/2 C
37% sol F, 0.5 g sol F, 0.9 g ins F, 1.4 tot g F, 63% ins F

Hominy, canned, 1/2 C
44% sol F, 0.9 g sol F, 1.2 g ins F, 2.1 tot g F, 56% ins F

Jicama, cooked, 1/2 C
42% sol F, 0.6 g sol F, 0.8 g ins F, 1.3 tot g F, 58% ins F

Jicama, raw, 1/2 C
53% sol F, 1.7 g sol F, 1.5 g ins F, 3.2 tot g F, 47% ins F

Kale, cooked, 1/2 C
28% sol F, 0.7 g sol F, 1.8 g ins F, 2.5 tot g F, 72% ins F

Kohlrabi, cooked, 1/2 C
67% sol F, 0.6 g sol F, 0.3 g ins F, 0.9 tot g F, 33% ins F

Kohlrabi, raw, 1/2 C
69% sol F, 1.7 g sol F, 0.8 g ins F, 2.5 tot g F, 31% ins F

Lentils, cooked, 1/2 C
16% sol F, 0.7 g sol F, 3.8 g ins F, 4.5 tot g F, 84% ins F

Lettuce, arugula, 1/2 C
Trace of sol F, 0.2 g ins F, 0.2 tot g F, 100% ins F

Lettuce, butterhead, 1/2 C
46% sol F, 0.3 g sol F, 0.4 g ins F, 0.7 tot g F, 54% ins F

Lettuce, chicory, 1/2 C
22% sol F, 0.1 g sol F, 0.5 g ins F, 0.6 tot g F, 78% ins F

Lettuce, endive, 1/2 C
21% sol F, 0.2 g sol F, 0.6 g ins F, 0.8 tot g F, 79% ins F

Lettuce, iceberg, 1/2 C
30% sol F, 0.2 g sol F, 0.4 g ins F, 0.5 tot g F, 70% ins F

Lettuce, radicchio, 1/2 C
19% sol F, 0.0 g sol F, 0.1 g ins F, 0.2 tot g F, 81% ins F

Lettuce, romaine, 1/2 C
43% sol F, 0.2 g sol F, 0.2 g ins F, 0.4 tot g F, 57% ins F

Miso (soybean paste), 1 tsp
33% sol F, 0.1 g sol F, 0.2 g ins F, 0.3 tot g F, 67% ins F

Mushrooms, cooked, fresh, 1/2 C
9% sol F, 0.2 g sol F, 1.6 g ins F, 1.7 tot g F, 91% ins F

Mushrooms, raw, pieces, 1/2 C
13% sol F, 0.1 g sol F, 0.4 g ins F, 0.4 tot g F, 88% ins F

Okra, fresh, cooked, 1/2 C
39% sol F, 1.0 g sol F, 1.6 g ins F, 2.6 tot g F, 61% ins F

Okra, frozen, cooked, 1/2 C
24% sol F, 1.0 g sol F, 3.1 g ins F, 4.1 tot g F, 76% ins F

Olives, black, 1 med
50% sol F, 0.1 g sol F, 0.1 g ins F, 0.2 tot g F, 50% ins F

Olives, green, 1 med
Trace of sol F, 0.1 g ins F, 0.1 tot g F, 100% ins F

Olives, stuffed, 1 med
Trace of sol F, 0.1 g ins F, 0.1 tot g F, 100% ins F

Onions, raw, chopped, 1/2 C
53% sol F, 0.9 g sol F, 0.8 g ins F, 1.7 tot g F, 47% ins F

Parsnips, cooked, 1/2 C
50% sol F, 2.0 g sol F, 2.0 g ins F, 4.0 tot g F, 50% ins F

Peas, blackeyed, 1/2 C
12% sol F, 0.5 g sol F, 3.6 g ins F, 4.1 tot g F, 88% ins F

Peas, chickpeas, cooked, 1/2 C
30% sol F, 1.3 g sol F, 3.0 g ins F, 4.3 tot g F, 70% ins F

Peas, cowpeas, dried, cooked, 1/2 C
13% sol F, 0.7 g sol F, 4.9 g ins F, 5.6 tot g F, 88% ins F

Peas, cowpeas, fresh, cooked, 1/2 C
11% sol F, 0.5 g sol F, 3.7 g ins F, 4.2 tot g F, 89% ins F

Peas, green, canned, 1/2 C
27% sol F, 0.9 g sol F, 2.3 g ins F, 3.2 tot g F, 73% ins F

Peas, green, cooked, 1/2 C
27% sol F, 1.2 g sol F, 3.2 g ins F, 4.4 tot g F, 73% ins F

Peas, green, frozen, cooked, 1/2 C
27% sol F, 1.2 g sol F, 3.1 g ins F, 4.3 tot g F, 73% ins F

Peas, pigeon, cooked, 1/2 C
17% sol F, 1.0 g sol F, 5.0 g ins F, 6.0 tot g F, 83% ins F

Peas, snow, cooked, 1/2 C
24% sol F, 1.1 g sol F, 3.4 g ins F, 4.5 tot g F, 76% ins F

Peas, split, dried, cooked, 1/2 C
13% sol F, 1.1 g sol F, 7.1 g ins F, 8.2 tot g F, 87% ins F

Peppers, green, raw, chopped, 1/2 C
38% sol F, 0.5 g sol F, 0.8 g ins F, 1.3 tot g F, 62% ins F

Peppers, green, cooked, 1/2 C
68% sol F, 0.8 g sol F, 0.4 g ins F, 1.1 tot g F, 32% ins F

Peppers, hot chili, green, cooked, 1/2 C
65% sol F, 0.7 g sol F, 0.4 g ins F, 1.0 tot g F, 35% ins F

Peppers, hot chili, green, raw, 1/2 C
39% sol F, 0.5 g sol F, 0.7 g ins F, 1.2 tot g F, 61% ins F

Peppers, hot chili, red, cooked, 1/2 C
38% sol F, 0.4 g sol F, 0.7 g ins F, 1.1 tot g F, 62% ins F

Peppers, hot chili, red, raw, 1/2 C
39% sol F, 0.5 g sol F, 0.7 g ins F, 1.2 tot g F, 61% ins F

Peppers, hot chili, sun-dried, 1/2 C
Trace of sol F, 5.3 g ins F, 5.3 tot g F, 100% ins F

Peppers, jalapeno, fresh, cooked, 1/2 C
38% sol F, 0.8 g sol F, 1.2 g ins F, 2.0 tot g F, 62% ins F

Peppers, jalapeno, fresh, raw, 1/2 C
40% sol F, 0.5 g sol F, 0.8 g ins F, 1.3 tot g F, 60% ins F

Peppers, red, cooked, 1/2 C
59% sol F, 0.7 g sol F, 0.5 g ins F, 1.1 tot g F, 41% ins F

Peppers, red, raw, chopped, 1/2 C
37% sol F, 0.6 g sol F, 1.0 g ins F, 1.5 tot g F, 63% ins F

Peppers, yellow, cooked, 1/2 C
35% sol F, 0.3 g sol F, 0.6 g ins F, 0.9 tot g F, 65% ins F

Peppers, yellow, raw, 1/2 C
38% sol F, 0.3 g sol F, 0.4 g ins F, 0.7 tot g F, 62% ins F

Pickles, bread and butter, 1/2 C
22% sol F, 0.2 g sol F, 0.7 g ins F, 0.9 tot g F, 78% ins F

Pickles, dill, 1/2 C
18% sol F, 0.2 g sol F, 0.7 g ins F, 0.9 tot g F, 82% ins F

Pickles, sweet gherkins, 1/2 C
24% sol F, 0.2 g sol F, 0.7 g ins F, 0.9 tot g F, 76% ins F

Potatoes, baked, with skin, 1 med
25% sol F, 1.0 g sol F, 3.0 g ins F, 4.0 tot g F, 75% ins F

Potatoes, baked, without skin, 1/2 C
68% sol F, 0.7 g sol F, 0.3 g ins F, 1.0 tot g F, 32% ins F

Potatoes, boiled, with skin, 1/2 C
40% sol F, 0.6 g sol F, 0.9 g ins F, 1.5 tot g F, 60% ins F

Potatoes, boiled, without skin, 1/2 C
57% sol F, 0.8 g sol F, 0.6 g ins F, 1.4 tot g F, 43% ins F

Potatoes, French fries, 100 g
56% sol F, 1.4 g sol F, 1.1 g ins F, 2.5 tot g F, 44% ins F

Potatoes, mashed, 1/2 C
56% sol F, 0.9 g sol F, 0.7 g ins F, 1.6 tot g F, 44% ins F

Potatoes, peeled, 1 med
56% sol F, 1.5 g sol F, 1.2 g ins F, 2.7 tot g F, 44% ins F

Potatoes, sweet, baked, 1/2 med
50% sol F, 1.0 g sol F, 1.0 g ins F, 2.0 tot g F, 50% ins F

Potatoes, sweet, flesh, cooked, 1/2 C
45% sol F, 1.8 g sol F, 2.2 g ins F, 4.0 tot g F, 55% ins F

Potatoes, sweet, French fries, 100 g
45% sol F, 1.6 g sol F, 1.9 g ins F, 3.5 tot g F, 55% ins F

Potatoes, sweet, peeled, 1 med
50% sol F, 1.7 g sol F, 1.7 g ins F, 3.4 tot g F, 50% ins F

Potatoes, with skin, 1 small
58% sol F, 2.2 g sol F, 1.6 g ins F, 3.8 tot g F, 42% ins F

Pumpkin, mashed, 1/2 C
14% sol F, 0.5 g sol F, 3.1 g ins F, 3.6 tot g F, 86% ins F

Radishes, 1/2 C
26% sol F, 0.3 g sol F, 0.7 g ins F, 1.0 tot g F, 74% ins F

Rutabagas, cooked, 1/2 C
16% sol F, 0.3 g sol F, 1.3 g ins F, 1.6 tot g F, 84% ins F

Sauerkraut, 1/2 C
34% sol F, 1.0 g sol F, 2.0 g ins F, 3.0 tot g F, 66% ins F

Scallions/spring onions, cooked, 1/2 C
53% sol F, 1.5 g sol F, 1.3 g ins F, 2.8 tot g F, 47% ins F

Scallions/spring onions, raw, 1/2 C
62% sol F, 0.8 g sol F, 0.5 g ins F, 1.3 tot g F, 38% ins F

Spinach, cooked, 1/2 C
33% sol F, 1.0 g sol F, 2.0 g ins F, 3.0 tot g F, 67% ins F

Spinach, raw, 1/2 C
25% sol F, 0.1 g sol F, 0.2 g ins F, 0.2 tot g F, 75% ins F

Squash, acorn, baked, 1/2 C
58% sol F, 2.3 g sol F, 1.7 g ins F, 4.0 tot g F, 43% ins F

Squash, butternut, cooked, 1/2 C
42% sol F, 0.7 g sol F, 1.0 g ins F, 1.7 tot g F, 58% ins F

Squash, chayote, cooked, 1/2 C
22% sol F, 0.5 g sol F, 1.8 g ins F, 2.3 tot g F, 78% ins F

Squash, Hubbard, cooked, 1/2 C
58% sol F, 1.9 g sol F, 1.4 g ins F, 3.3 tot g F, 42% ins F

Squash, spaghetti, cooked, 1/2 C
55% sol F, 0.6 g sol F, 0.5 g ins F, 1.1 tot g F, 45% ins F

Squash, summer, cooked, 1/2 C
48% sol F, 1.1 g sol F, 1.2 g ins F, 2.3 tot g F, 52% ins F

Squash, winter, cooked, 1/2 C
67% sol F, 2.0 g sol F, 1.0 g ins F, 3.0 tot g F, 33% ins F

Squash, zucchini, cooked, 1/2 C
44% sol F, 0.6 g sol F, 0.7 g ins F, 1.3 tot g F, 56% ins F

Tempeh (fermented soy cake), 1 oz
45% sol F, 1.3 g sol F, 1.6 g ins F, 2.9 tot g F, 55% ins F

Textured soy protein, from dry, 1/2 C
28% sol F, 1.3 g sol F, 3.3 g ins F, 4.6 tot g F, 72% ins F

Tofu, 1/2 C
50% sol F, 0.2 g sol F, 0.2 g ins F, 0.4 tot g F, 50% ins F

Tomato juice, 1/2 C
50% sol F, 0.3 g sol F, 0.3 g ins F, 0.5 tot g F, 50% ins F

Tomato paste, 1/2 C
20% sol F, 1.1 g sol F, 4.3 g ins F, 5.4 tot g F, 80% ins F

Tomato puree, 1/2 C
40% sol F, 1.0 g sol F, 1.5 g ins F, 2.5 tot g F, 60% ins F

Tomato sauce, 1/2 C
47% sol F, 0.8 g sol F, 0.9 g ins F, 1.7 tot g F, 53% ins F

Tomatoes, canned, 1/2 C
38% sol F, 0.5 g sol F, 0.8 g ins F, 1.3 tot g F, 62% ins F

Tomatoes, green, raw, 1/2 C
10% sol F, 0.1 g sol F, 0.9 g ins F, 1.0 tot g F, 90% ins F

Tomatoes, orange, raw, 1/2 C
7% sol F, 0.1 g sol F, 0.7 g ins F, 0.7 tot g F, 93% ins F

Tomatoes, red, raw, 1/2 C
10% sol F, 0.1 g sol F, 0.9 g ins F, 1.0 tot g F, 90% ins F

Tomatoes, raw, 1/2 C
13% sol F, 0.1 g sol F, 0.8 g ins F, 0.9 tot g F, 87% ins F

Tomatoes, sun-dried, dry-pack, 1/2 C
9% sol F, 0.3 g sol F, 3.0 g ins F, 3.3 tot g F, 91% ins F

Tomatoes, sun-dried, oil-pack, 1/2 C
9% sol F, 0.3 g sol F, 2.9 g ins F, 3.2 tot g F, 91% ins F

Tomatoes, yellow, raw, 1/2 C
10% sol F, 0.1 g sol F, 0.5 g ins F, 0.5 tot g F, 90% ins F

Tomatilloes, raw, 1/2 C
8% sol F, 0.1 g sol F, 1.2 g ins F, 1.3 tot g F, 92% ins F

Turnip greens, cooked, 1/2 C
44% sol F, 1.1 g sol F, 1.4 g ins F, 2.5 tot g F, 56% ins F

Turnips, cooked, 1/2 C
50% sol F, 1.0 g sol F, 1.0 g ins F, 2.0 tot g F, 50% ins F

Vegetable juice, V-8, 1/2 C
29% sol F, 0.2 g sol F, 0.5 g ins F, 0.7 tot g F, 71% ins F

Watercress, 1/2 C
Trace of sol F, 0.1 g ins F, 0.1 tot g F, 100% ins F

Yams, cooked, 1/2 C
37% sol F, 1.4 g sol F, 2.4 g ins F, 3.8 tot g F, 63% ins F

Zucchini, cooked, 1/2 C
44% sol F, 1.1 g sol F, 1.4 g ins F, 2.5 tot g F, 56% ins F

Nuts and Seeds

Almond butter, 1 Tbsp
17% sol F, 0.1 g sol F, 0.5 g ins F, 0.6 tot g F, 83% ins F

Almond paste, 1 Tbsp
13% sol F, 0.1 g sol F, 0.7 g ins F, 0.8 tot g F, 88% ins F

Almonds, 1/4 C
10% sol F, 0.4 g sol F, 3.5 g ins F, 3.9 tot g F, 90% ins F

Brazil nuts, 1 Tbsp
20% sol F, 0.1 g sol F, 0.4 g ins F, 0.5 tot g F, 80% ins F

Cashews, 1/4 C
55% sol F, 0.6 g sol F, 0.5 g ins F, 1.1 tot g F, 45% ins F

Chestnuts, 1/4 C
21% sol F, 0.9 g sol F, 3.3 g ins F, 4.2 tot g F, 79% ins F

Coconut, dried, 1.5 Tbsp
7% sol F, 0.1 g sol F, 1.4 g ins F, 1.5 tot g F, 93% ins F

Coconut, raw, 2 Tbsp
9% sol F, 0.1 g sol F, 1.0 g ins F, 1.1 tot g F, 91% ins F

Filberts, raw, 10 nuts
Trace of sol F, 1.0 g ins F, 1.0 tot g F, 100% ins F

Flax seeds, 1/4 C
54% sol F, 3.5 g sol F, 2.9 g ins F, 6.4 tot g F, 46% ins F

Hazelnuts, 1 Tbsp
40% sol F, 0.2 g sol F, 0.3 g ins F, 0.5 tot g F, 60% ins F

Hickory nuts, 1/4 C
23% sol F, 0.5 g sol F, 1.5 g ins F, 1.9 tot g F, 77% ins F

Macadamia nuts, 1/4 C
21% sol F, 0.7 g sol F, 2.5 g ins F, 3.1 tot g F, 79% ins F

Peanut butter, chunky, 1 Tbsp
15% sol F, 0.2 g sol F, 1.1 g ins F, 1.3 tot g F, 85% ins F

Peanut butter, smooth, 1 Tbsp
30% sol F, 0.3 g sol F, 0.7 g ins F, 1.0 tot g F, 70% ins F

Peanuts, dry roasted, 1/4 C
28% sol F, 0.7 g sol F, 1.8 g ins F, 2.5 tot g F, 72% ins F

Pecans, 1/4 C
20% sol F, 0.4 g sol F, 1.7 g ins F, 2.1 tot g F, 80% ins F

Pine nuts/pignolias, 1/4 C
10% sol F, 0.4 g sol F, 3.3 g ins F, 3.7 tot g F, 90% ins F

Pine nuts/pinyon, 1/4 C
10% sol F, 0.4 g sol F, 3.1 g ins F, 3.5 tot g F, 90% ins F

Pistachio nuts, 1/4 C
25% sol F, 0.9 g sol F, 2.6 g ins F, 3.5 tot g F, 75% ins F

Poppy seeds, 1/4 C
Trace of sol F, 3.5 g ins F, 3.5 tot g F, 100% ins F

Pumpkin seeds, 1/4 C
27% sol F, 0.6 g sol F, 1.6 g ins F, 2.2 tot g F, 73% ins F

Sesame butter/tahini, 1 Tbsp
21% sol F, 0.3 g sol F, 1.1 g ins F, 1.4 tot g F, 79% ins F

Sesame seeds, 1/4 C
21% sol F, 0.7 g sol F, 2.6 g ins F, 3.3 tot g F, 79% ins F

Squash seeds, 1/4 C
27% sol F, 0.6 g sol F, 1.6 g ins F, 2.2 tot g F, 73% ins F

Sunflower butter, 1 Tbsp
38% sol F, 0.5 g sol F, 0.8 g ins F, 1.3 tot g F, 62% ins F

Sunflower seeds, 1/4 C
32% sol F, 0.7 g sol F, 1.5 g ins F, 2.2 tot g F, 68% ins F

Walnuts, 1/4 C
36% sol F, 0.5 g sol F, 0.9 g ins F, 1.4 tot g F, 64% ins F

Water chestnuts, 1/4 C
75% sol F, 0.5 g sol F, 0.2 g ins F, 0.6 tot g F, 25% ins F

Fruits

Apples, dried, 1/2 C
55% sol F, 2.1 g sol F, 1.7 g ins F, 3.8 tot g F, 45% ins F

Apples, raw, w/skin, 1 med
36% sol F, 1.5 g sol F, 2.7 g ins F, 4.2 tot g F, 64% ins F

Applesauce, canned, 1/2 C
50% sol F, 1.0 g sol F, 1.0 g ins F, 2.0 tot g F, 50% ins F

Apricots, canned, 4 halves
42% sol F, 0.5 g sol F, 0.7 g ins F, 1.2 tot g F, 58% ins F

Apricots, dried, 5 halves
50% sol F, 1.0 g sol F, 1.0 g ins F, 2.0 tot g F, 50% ins F

Apricots, raw, 2 med
69% sol F, 0.9 g sol F, 0.4 g ins F, 1.3 tot g F, 31% ins F

Avocado, raw, 1/8
42% sol F, 0.5 g sol F, 0.7 g ins F, 1.2 tot g F, 58% ins F

Bananas, 1 small
50% sol F, 1.0 g sol F, 1.0 g ins F, 2.0 tot g F, 50% ins F

Bananas, 1 med
50% sol F, 1.5 g sol F, 1.5 g ins F, 3.0 tot g F, 50% ins F

Bananas, 1 large
50% sol F, 2.0 g sol F, 2.0 g ins F, 4.0 tot g F, 50% ins F

Black currant juice, 1/2 C
67% sol F, 0.5 g sol F, 0.3 g ins F, 0.8 tot g F, 33% ins F

Blackberries, raw, 1/2 C
19% sol F, 0.7 g sol F, 3.0 g ins F, 3.7 tot g F, 81% ins F

Blueberries, raw, 1/2 C
20% sol F, 0.4 g sol F, 1.6 g ins F, 2.0 tot g F, 80% ins F

Cantaloupe, 1/4 med
Trace of sol F, 1.0 g ins F, 1.0 tot g F, 100% ins F

Cherries, raw, 1/2 C
29% sol F, 0.5 g sol F, 1.2 g ins F, 1.7 tot g F, 71% ins F

Cherries, canned, 12 large
46% sol F, 0.6 g sol F, 0.7 g ins F, 1.3 tot g F, 54% ins F

Cherries, maraschino, 1/2 C
29% sol F, 0.2 g sol F, 0.5 g ins F, 0.7 tot g F, 71% ins F

Cranberries, dried, 1/2 C
27% sol F, 0.8 g sol F, 2.2 g ins F, 3.0 tot g F, 73% ins F

Cranberries, fresh, 1/2 C
25% sol F, 0.5 g sol F, 1.5 g ins F, 2.0 tot g F, 75% ins F

Cranberry juice, 1/2 C
33% sol F, 0.1 g sol F, 0.1 g ins F, 0.2 tot g F, 67% ins F

Currants, dried, 2 Tbsp
50% sol F, 0.2 g sol F, 0.2 g ins F, 0.4 tot g F, 50% ins F

Dates, 3 fruits
Trace of sol F, 2.0 g ins F, 2.0 tot g F, 100% ins F

Elderberries, 1/2 C
19% sol F, 1.0 g sol F, 4.2 g ins F, 5.1 tot g F, 81% ins F

Figs, dried, 3 ea
43% sol F, 2.0 g sol F, 2.6 g ins F, 4.6 tot g F, 57% ins F

Fruit cocktail, canned, 1/2 C
35% sol F, 0.7 g sol F, 1.3 g ins F, 2.0 tot g F, 65% ins F

Gooseberries, 1/2 C
22% sol F, 0.7 g sol F, 2.6 g ins F, 3.3 tot g F, 78% ins F

Grapefruit, 1/2 med
69% sol F, 0.9 g sol F, 0.4 g ins F, 1.3 tot g F, 31% ins F

Grapes, raw, w/skin, 1/2 C
38% sol F, 0.3 g sol F, 0.5 g ins F, 0.8 tot g F, 63% ins F

Guava, raw, ripe, 100 g
12% sol F, 1.5 g sol F, 11.2 g ins F, 12.7 tot g F, 88% ins F

Kiwifruits, raw, flesh only, 1 large
41% sol F, 0.7 g sol F, 1.0 g ins F, 1.7 tot g F, 59% ins F

Kiwifruits, raw, w/skin, 1 large
70% sol F, 0.7 g sol F, 0.3 g ins F, 1.0 tot g F, 30% ins F

Kumquats, 1 med
38% sol F, 0.5 g sol F, 0.8 g ins F, 1.3 tot g F, 62% ins F

Lemons, 1 med
63% sol F, 1.0 g sol F, 0.6 g ins F, 1.6 tot g F, 38% ins F

Loganberries, 1/2 C
10% sol F, 0.4 g sol F, 3.3 g ins F, 3.6 tot g F, 90% ins F

Mangoes, raw, flesh only, 1/2 small
59% sol F, 1.7 g sol F, 1.2 g ins F, 2.9 tot g F, 41% ins F

Mangoes, raw, flesh and skin, 100 g
39% sol F, 0.7 g sol F, 1.1 g ins F, 1.8 tot g F, 61% ins F

Melons, cantaloupe, cubed, 1/2 C
27% sol F, 0.2 g sol F, 0.4 g ins F, 0.6 tot g F, 73% ins F

Melons, honeydew, 1/2 C
33% sol F, 0.2 g sol F, 0.3 g ins F, 0.5 tot g F, 67% ins F

Melons, watermelon, cubed, 1/2 C
67% sol F, 0.2 g sol F, 0.1 g ins F, 0.2 tot g F, 33% ins F

Nectarines, 1 small
44% sol F, 0.8 g sol F, 1.0 g ins F, 1.8 tot g F, 56% ins F

Oranges, 1 med
64% sol F, 1.6 g sol F, 0.9 g ins F, 2.5 tot g F, 36% ins F

Oranges, mandarin, 1/2 C
40% sol F, 0.9 g sol F, 1.4 g ins F, 2.3 tot g F, 60% ins F

Papayas, cubed, 1/2 C
60% sol F, 0.8 g sol F, 0.5 g ins F, 1.3 tot g F, 40% ins F

Papaya juice, 1/2 C
47% sol F, 0.4 g sol F, 0.4 g ins F, 0.8 tot g F, 53% ins F

Passion fruit, purple, fresh, 1 med
74% sol F, 1.4 g sol F, 0.5 g ins F, 1.9 tot g F, 26% ins F

Peach nectar (juice), 1/2 C
73% sol F, 0.6 g sol F, 0.2 g ins F, 0.8 tot g F, 27% ins F

Peaches, canned, drained, 1/2 C
50% sol F, 1.0 g sol F, 1.0 g ins F, 2.0 tot g F, 50% ins F

Peaches, dried, 1/2 C
47% sol F, 3.1 g sol F, 3.5 g ins F, 6.6 tot g F, 53% ins F

Peaches, dried, cooked, 1/2 C
46% sol F, 1.6 g sol F, 1.9 g ins F, 3.5 tot g F, 54% ins F

Peaches, raw, flesh only, 100 g
45% sol F, 0.9 g sol F, 1.1 g ins F, 2.0 tot g F, 55% ins F

Peaches, raw, w/skin, 1 med
40% sol F, 1.3 g sol F, 1.9 g ins F, 3.2 tot g F, 60% ins F

Peaches, raw, w/skin, 100 g
40% sol F, 1.2 g sol F, 1.7 g ins F, 2.9 tot g F, 60% ins F

Pears, canned, drained, per half
33% sol F, 0.4 g sol F, 0.8 g ins F, 1.2 tot g F, 67% ins F

Pears, dried, 1/2 C
40% sol F, 2.7 g sol F, 4.1 g ins F, 6.8 tot g F, 60% ins F

Pears, dried, cooked, 1/2 C
54% sol F, 4.4 g sol F, 3.8 g ins F, 8.2 tot g F, 46% ins F

Pears, raw, w/skin, 1 med
11% sol F, 0.5 g sol F, 4.0 g ins F, 4.5 tot g F, 89% ins F

Persimmons, 1 med
13% sol F, 0.8 g sol F, 5.3 g ins F, 6.1 tot g F, 87% ins F

Pineapple, canned, 1/3 C
14% sol F, 0.2 g sol F, 1.2 g ins F, 1.4 tot g F, 86% ins F

Pineapple, raw, 1/2 C
11% sol F, 0.1 g sol F, 0.9 g ins F, 1.0 tot g F, 89% ins F

Plaintains, 1/2 C
20% sol F, 0.4 g sol F, 1.4 g ins F, 1.8 tot g F, 80% ins F

Plums, raw, 5 small
50% sol F, 2.0 g sol F, 2.0 g ins F, 4.0 tot g F, 50% ins F

Pomegranates, 1 med
20% sol F, 0.2 g sol F, 0.8 g ins F, 1.0 tot g F, 80% ins F

Prune juice, 1/2 C
53% sol F, 0.8 g sol F, 0.7 g ins F, 1.5 tot g F, 47% ins F

Prunes, cooked, 1/2 C
26% sol F, 2.1 g sol F, 6.1 g ins F, 8.2 tot g F, 74% ins F

Prunes, dried, 3 med
53% sol F, 1.0 g sol F, 0.9 g ins F, 1.9 tot g F, 47% ins F

Raisins, 1/4 C
27% sol F, 0.4 g sol F, 1.1 g ins F, 1.5 tot g F, 73% ins F

Raspberries, 1/2 C
11% sol F, 0.5 g sol F, 3.6 g ins F, 4.0 tot g F, 89% ins F

Rhubarb, cooked, sweetened, 1/2 C
25% sol F, 0.6 g sol F, 1.8 g ins F, 2.4 tot g F, 75% ins F

Rhubarb, cooked, unsweetened, 1/2 C
35% sol F, 0.6 g sol F, 1.1 g ins F, 1.7 tot g F, 65% ins F

Sapodillas, 1 med
35% sol F, 4.9 g sol F, 9.0 g ins F, 13.9 tot g F, 65% ins F

Starfruit (carambola), 1/2 C
45% sol F, 0.7 g sol F, 0.8 g ins F, 1.5 tot g F, 55% ins F

Strawberries, raw, 1/2 C
38% sol F, 0.6 g sol F, 1.0 g ins F, 1.6 tot g F, 63% ins F

Tangerines, 1 med
88% sol F, 1.4 g sol F, 0.2 g ins F, 1.6 tot g F, 13% ins F

Misc. & Supplements

Carob powder, 1 tsp
78% sol F, 0.7 g sol F, 0.2 g ins F, 0.9 tot g F, 22% ins F

Chocolate, baking, 1 oz
5% sol F, 0.2 g sol F, 4.2 g ins F, 4.4 tot g F, 95% ins F

Chocolate, dark, 1 oz
6% sol F, 0.1 g sol F, 1.6 g ins F, 1.7 tot g F, 94% ins F

Cocoa powder, unsweetened, 1 tsp
17% sol F, 0.1 g sol F, 0.5 g ins F, 0.6 tot g F, 83% ins F

Corn chips, 1/2 C
Trace of sol F, 0.6 g ins F, 0.6 tot g F, 100% ins F

Corn nuts, 1/2 C
2% sol F, 0.1 g sol F, 2.9 g ins F, 2.9 tot g F, 98% ins F

Halvah, plain, 1 oz
23% sol F, 0.3 g sol F, 1.0 g ins F, 1.3 tot g F, 77% ins F

Kashi soft-baked bars, 1 bar
33% sol F, 1.0 g sol F, 2.0 g ins F, 3.0 tot g F, 67% ins F

Licorice, 1 oz
50% sol F, 0.2 g sol F, 0.2 g ins F, 0.4 tot g F, 50% ins F

Mott's Fruitsations, all flavors, 111 g (1/2 C)
50% sol F, 0.5 g sol F, 0.5 g ins F, 1.0 tot g F, 50% ins F

Potato chips, 1 oz
57% sol F, 0.8 g sol F, 0.6 g ins F, 1.4 tot g F, 43% ins F

Pretzels, 1 oz
27% sol F, 0.3 g sol F, 0.8 g ins F, 1.1 tot g F, 73% ins F

Supp, Benefibre, rounded tsp
100% sol F, 3.0 g sol F, 0.0 g ins F, 3.0 tot g F, 0% ins F

Supp, Citrucel, 4 capsules
100% sol F, 2.0 g sol F, 0.0 g ins F, 2.0 tot g F, 0% ins F

Supp, Konsyl Original Fiber, 1 tsp
50% sol F, 3.0 g sol F, 3.0 g ins F, 6.0 tot g F, 50% ins F

Supp, Metamucil, 1 tsp
59% sol F, 2.0 g sol F, 1.4 g ins F, 3.4 tot g F, 41% ins F

Supp, Yarrow Gentle Fibers, 2 Tbsp
33% sol F, 3.0 g sol F, 6.0 g ins F, 9.0 tot g F, 67% ins F

Supp, Yerba Prima Fiber, 4 capsules
82% sol F, 1.8 g sol F, 0.4 g ins F, 2.2 tot g F, 18% ins F

Foods with a High Soluble:Insoluble Fiber Ratio

Note: These are fiber ratios.

For example, psyllium husk has a total of 8 grams of fiber per 10 grams. Of that fiber, 89% (or 7.1 grams) is soluble.

Knowing the percentage allows you to look at a food label and estimate the soluble fiber by multiplying the total fiber times the percentage. This is not an exact science, but it will definitely help you make the right fiber decisions.

If anything is a trigger for you, please avoid it.

Flour, konjac—100%
Supp, Benefibre—100%
Supp, Citrucel—100%
Flour, cornstarch—93%
Psyllium husk—89%
Tangerines—88%
Supp, Yerba Prima Fiber—82%
Carob powder—78%
Water chestnuts—75%
Passion fruit, purple, fresh—74%
Peach nectar (juice)—73%
Artichokes—72%
Kiwifruits, raw, w/skin—70%
Kohlrabi, raw—69%
Apricots, raw—69%
Grapefruit—69%
Potatoes, baked, without skin—68%
Peppers, green, cooked—68%
Bread, buns, sourdough—67%
Melons, watermelon, cubed—67%
Black currant juice—67%
Brussels sprouts, cooked—67%
Kohlrabi, cooked—67%
Squash, winter, cooked—67%
Oatmeal, instant, cooked—66%

Peppers, hot chili, green, cooked—65%
Oranges—64%
Bread, matzo/matzah, egg—63%
Lemons—63%
Collard greens, raw—62%
Scallions/spring onions, raw—62%
Asparagus, cooked—61%
Collard greens, cooked—60%
Biscuits, baking powder, buttermilk—60%
Bread, buns, crescent (refrig dough)—60%
Bread, cheese—60%
Bread, Italian—60%
Papayas, cubed—60%
Sprouts, mung bean, cooked—60%
Peppers, red, cooked—59%
Supp, Metamucil—59%
Mangoes, raw, flesh only—59%
Bread, buns, French—58%
Bread, buns, Vienna—58%
Bread, focaccia—58%
Potatoes, with skin—58%
Squash, Hubbard, cooked—58%
Squash, acorn, baked—58%
Sprouts, acorn, cooked—57%
Potato chips—57%
Potatoes, boiled, without skin—57%
Potatoes, mashed—56%
Potatoes, French fries—56%
Flour, oat—56%
Potatoes, peeled—56%
Oat bran, cooked—55%
Apples, dried—55%
Bread, buns, oatmeal—55%
Cashews—55%
Squash, spaghetti, cooked—55%

Foods with a High Insoluble:Soluble Fiber Ratio

Note once again, these are fiber ratios.

For example, cornflakes, part of a low-residue diet, have a total of 0.4 grams of fiber per 1/2 cup. Of that fiber, almost 100% is insoluble.

Knowing the percentage allows you to look at a food label and estimate the insoluble fiber by multiplying the total fiber times the percentage. This is not an exact science, but it will definitely help you make the right fiber decisions.

If anything is a trigger for you, please avoid it.

Bran Chex, Multi—100%
Bran Flakes, without raisins—100%
Bran, wheat, dry—100%
Bread, multigrain or granola—100%
Cantaloupe—100%
Complete Bran Flakes—100%
Corn chips—100%
Cornflakes—100%
Cracked Wheat, cooked—100%
Crackers, graham—100%
Cracklin' Oat Bran—100%
Dates—100%
Filberts, raw—100%
Flour, teff—100%
Grape-Nuts Flakes—100%
Just Right Fruit and Nut—100%
Kashi 7 Whole Grain Puffed Cereal —100%
Lettuce, arugula—100%
Nature's Path Organic Corn Flakes—100%
Nature's Path Organic Crispy Rice—100%
Nutri-Grain-Golden Wheat—100%
Olives, green—100%
Olives, stuffed—100%
Pasta, spaghetti, cooked—100%

Peppers, hot chili, sun-dried—100%
Poppy seeds—100%
Smacks—100%
Smart Start—100%
Watercress—100%
Wheat, gluten—100%
Cornmeal, dry—99%
Corn nuts—98%
Flour, arrowroot—98%
Bran, corn, dry—97%
Wafers, rye—97%
Corn Bran—97%
Cornmeal, cooked—96%
Flour, barley bran—96%
Chocolate, baking—95%
Chocolate, dark—94%
Coconut, dried—93%
Fiber One—93%
Tomatoes, orange, raw—93%
All-Bran—92%
All-Bran with Extra Fiber—92%
Tomatilloes, raw—92%
100% Bran—92%
Mushrooms, cooked, fresh—91%
Coconut, raw—91%
Tomatoes, sun-dried, dry-pack—91%
Tomatoes, sun-dried, oil-pack—91%
Beans, white, cooked—90%
Loganberries—90%
Pasta, No Yolks, cooked—90%
Tomatoes, green, raw—90%
Tomatoes, red, raw—90%
Tomatoes, yellow, raw—90%
Pine nuts/pinyon—90%
Almonds—90%
Pine nuts/pignolias—90%
Pineapple, raw—89%
Bread, buns, hamburger, WW—89%
Peas, cowpeas, fresh, cooked—89%

Beans, kidney, cooked—89%
Pancakes—89%
Pears, raw, w/skin—89%
Rice, brown, cooked—89%
Raspberries—89%
Muffins, bran—88%
Wheat, spelt—88%
Guava, raw, ripe—88%
Peas, blackeyed—88%
Almond paste—88%
Corn, whole kernel, canned—88%
Mushrooms, raw, pieces—88%
Peas, cowpeas, dried, cooked—88%
Broccoli, raw—87%
Bran, rice, dry—87%
Quinoa, cooked—87%
Corn, cooked—87%
Tomatoes, raw—87%
Persimmons—87%
Kasha, cooked—87%
Bread, bran—87%
Peas, split, dried, cooked—87%
Buckwheat groats, dry—86%
Pumpkin, mashed—86%
Quinoa, dry—86%
Flour, buckwheat—86%
Flour, WW—86%
Shredded Wheat—86%
Pineapple, canned—86%
Total Raisin Bran—85%
Flour, rice, brown—85%
Bread, flat, tortillas—85%
Pasta, spiral, cooked—85%
Peanut butter, chunky—85%
Rice, wild, cooked—85%
Lentils, cooked—84%
Flour, cornmeal, degermed—84%
Bread, pita, WW—84%
Bread, buns, WW—84%

Rolled wheat, cooked—84%
Rutabagas, cooked—84%
Chard, cooked—84%
Peas, pigeon, cooked—83%
Raisin Bran—83%
Almond butter—83%
Cocoa powder, unsweetened—83%
Muffins, corn—83%
Wheat, sprouted—83%
Bulgur, dry—83%
Pickles, dill—82%
Millet, cooked—82%
Muffins, English, WW—82%
Flour, triticale, whole grain—82%
Elderberries—81%
Millet, dry—81%
Blackberries, raw—81%
Pasta, spiral, WW, cooked—81%
Lettuce, radicchio—81%
Pecans—80%
Tomato paste—80%
Blueberries, raw—80%
Brazil nuts—80%
Kashi Heart to Heart—80%
Plaintains—80%
Pomegranates—80%
Wheat Chex—80%
Lettuce, endive—79%
Macadamia nuts—79%
Chestnuts—79%
Beans, chick beans, cooked—79%
Beans, garbanzo, cooked—79%
Flour, chickpea—79%
Sesame seeds—79%
Bread, cornbread—79%
Sesame butter/tahini—79%
Gooseberries—78%
Flour, barley malt—78%
Barley, dry—78%

Flour, barley—78%
Couscous, dry—78%
Celery, raw, chopped—78%
Couscous, cooked—78%
Crackers, melba—78%
Pasta, rice noodles, cooked—78%
Pickles, bread and butter—78%
Special K—78%
Squash, chayote, cooked—78%
Lettuce, chicory—78%
Bread, WW—77%
Halvah, plain—77%
Hickory nuts—77%
Pickles, sweet gherkins—76%
Bread, Boston brown—76%
Okra, frozen, cooked—76%
Peas, snow, cooked—76%
Pistachio nuts—75%
Barley, cooked—75%
Beans, green, canned—75%
Beans, northern, cooked—75%
Bran Buds—75%
Bread, oatmeal—75%
Bread, raisin—75%
Bulger, cooked—75%
Bulgur, cooked—75%
Cheerios—75%
Crackers, Wheat Thins—75%
Cranberries, fresh—75%
Cream of rice, cooked—75%
Cucumbers—75%
Eggplants—75%
Mueslix—75%
Original Frosted Mini-Wheats—75%
Pasta, spaghetti, WW, cooked—75%
Potatoes, baked, with skin—75%
Rhubarb, cooked, sweetened—75%
Spinach, raw—75%
Sprouts, alfalfa, raw—75%

Total—75%
Wheat Germ, RTE—75%
Prunes, cooked—74%
Beans, pinto, cooked—74%
Carrot juice—74%
Radishes—74%
Bread, buns, brown—73%
Bread, buns, cracked wheat—73%
Bread, buns, multigrain—73%
Cranberries, dried—73%
Muffins, English, white—73%
Raisins—73%
Flour, rye—73%
Peas, green, canned—73%
Peas, green, frozen, cooked—73%
Melons, cantaloupe, cubed—73%
Peas, green, cooked—73%
Pretzels—73%
Pumpkin seeds—73%
Squash seeds—73%
Flour, peanut, low fat—73%
Bread, buns, hamburger, brown—72%
Kale, cooked—72%
Peanuts, dry roasted—72%
Textured soy protein, from dry—72%
Beet greens, raw—71%
Bread, buns, hoagie—71%
Bread, flat, corn tortillas—71%
Cherries, maraschino—71%
Popcorn, popped—71%
Rice, white, instant, cooked—71%
Vegetable juice, V-8—71%
Bread, bagels, WW—71%
Cherries, raw—71%
Bread, cracked wheat—70%
Cauliflower, cooked—70%
Lettuce, iceberg—70%
Peanut butter, smooth—70%
Sorghum—70%

Peas, chickpeas, cooked—70%
Oats, whole, cooked—69%
Amaranth, dry—68%
Sunflower seeds—68%
Corn grits, cooked—68%
Bread, sourdough—68%
Bread, bagels, oat bran—67%
Flour, rice, white—67%
Basic 4—67%
Beans, navy, cooked—67%
Bran, oat, dry—67%
Cheerios, Multigrain—67%
Complete Oat Bran Flakes—67%
Granola, low fat with raisins—67%
Kashi soft-baked bars—67%
Melons, honeydew—67%
Spinach, cooked—67%
Supp, Yarrow Gentle Fibers—67%
Bread, buns, hamburger, white—67%
Bread, buns, hard—67%
Bread, buns, hot dog, white—67%
Bread, buns, kaiser—67%
Bread, Hovis—67%
Crackers, saltine—67%
Cranberry juice—67%
Miso (soybean paste)—67%
Pears, canned, drained—67%
Rice Krispies—67%
Rice, white, cooked—67%
Sauerkraut—66%
Fruit cocktail, canned—65%
Sapodillas—65%
Peppers, yellow, cooked—65%
Rhubarb, cooked, unsweetened—65%
Apples, raw, w/skin—64%
Walnuts—64%
Cauliflower, raw—64%
Flour, quinoa—64%
Bread, buns, white—64%

Bread, oat bran—64%
Cream of Wheat, uncooked—64%
Peppers, red, raw, chopped—63%
Yams, cooked—63%
Bok choy/pak choi, cooked—63%
Fennel bulb, raw—63%
Bread, bagels, white—63%
Bread, dinner rolls, white—63%
Grapes, raw, w/skin—63%
Pasta, egg noodles, cooked—63%
Sprouts, bean, raw—63%
Strawberries, raw—63%
Peppers, hot chili, red, cooked—62%
Beans, green/string canned—62%
Kumquats—62%
Peppers, green, raw, chopped—62%
Peppers, yellow, raw—62%
Sunflower butter—62%
Tomatoes, canned—62%
Peppers, jalapeno, fresh, cooked—62%
Bread, flour tortillas (wheat), RTE—61%
Asparagus, raw—61%
Beans, butter, cooked—61%
Peppers, hot chili, green, raw—61%
Peppers, hot chili, red, raw—61%
Mangoes, raw, flesh and skin—61%
Okra, fresh, cooked—61%
Beans, black, cooked—61%
Beans, bayo, cooked—60%
Beans, green, cooked—60%
Bread, French—60%
Bread, white—60%
Cassava (yuca), cooked—60%
Crackers, Ritz—60%
Crackers, Triscuits—60%
Hazelnuts—60%
Oranges, mandarin—60%
Peaches, raw, w/skin—60%
Pears, dried—60%

Peppers, jalapeno, fresh, raw—60%
Potatoes, boiled, with skin—60%
Tomato puree—60%
Peaches, raw, w/skin—60%
Kiwifruits, raw, flesh only—59%
Apricots, canned—58%
Avocado, raw—58%
Carrots, raw—58%
Jicama, cooked—58%
Squash, butternut, cooked—58%
Beans, lima, cooked—57%
Bok choy/pak choi, raw—57%
Lettuce, romaine—57%
Scones—57%
Waffles, round, 4-in diameter—57%
Cabbage, red, cooked—57%
Oats, rolled, cooked—57%
Figs, dried—57%
Hominy, canned—56%
Squash, zucchini, cooked—56%
Turnip greens, cooked—56%
Zucchini, cooked—56%
Flour, corn—56%
Cabbage, green, cooked—56%
Broccoflower, cooked—56%
Beets, raw, w/o skin—56%
Bread, rye—56%
Cabbage, green, raw—56%
Cabbage, red, raw—56%
Flour, soy—56%
Muffins, blueberry—56%
Nectarines—56%
Starfruit (carambola)—55%
Tempeh (fermented soy cake)—55%
Peaches, raw, flesh only—55%
Potatoes, sweet, flesh, cooked—55%
Potatoes, sweet, French fries—55%
Beans, soy, cooked—55%
Flour, soy, defatted—55%

Beet greens, cooked—55%

How Does Soluble Fiber Help IBS and IBD?

According to WebMD, soluble fiber relieves abdominal pain and discomfort in some people suffering from IBS.

"But how?" you may ask. "How does soluble fiber improve bowel symptoms?"

Soluble fiber is not digested by the body. It attracts water and forms a gel-like substance that helps to bulk up and soften the stool. It also slows digestion. This gel slides easily through an irritated intestinal tract, allowing everything (including hemorrhoids) to settle and heal.

East Tennessee Children's Hospital reports that soluble fiber is beneficial for IBD because it doesn't produce the type of particles that adhere to the bowel wall and cause inflammation.

This is great news for anyone with intestinal irritation.

Added benefits include lowering of cholesterol and regulation of blood-glucose levels.

Conversely, insoluble fiber speeds the passage of stool through the body. It makes IBS and IBD symptoms worse for many people. The Mayo Clinic states that it may be beneficial to limit insoluble fiber when you are experiencing an IBS episode. Inflammatory bowel disease sufferers are also advised to limit their intake of insoluble fiber and to consume a low-residue diet, especially during a flare-up or following surgery.

According to *IBS for Dummies*, anyone with IBS should eat lots of soluble fiber and avoid insoluble fiber, which is much tougher on the digestive system due to rough edges that may irritate sensitive intestines. The book states further that soluble fiber helps to trap water, which helps with diarrhea. Soluble fiber also softens hardening stool. This helps to relieve constipation.

However, you need both types of fiber.

The National Institute of Health recommends that you consume plenty if fluids while you increase dietary fiber *gradually*. This helps to avoid flatulence, bloating, and abdominal cramps. Once your body becomes accustomed to the increased fiber intake, you will be able to process it without uncomfortable side-effects.

Some studies indicate that the prebiotics in soluble fiber help your body digest probiotic supplements and foods like yogurt. Prebiotics feed the friendly probiotic bacteria, allowing it to grow and flourish. This process suppresses bad bacteria and yeast that may cause some of your symptoms.

Soluble fiber worked like a miracle for me. Temporarily, I had to give up some of my favorite foods like twelve-grain bread, salads, cherries, and baked potatoes with crusty skins. Every time I ignored common sense and tried something I shouldn't have, I paid the price.

Suggested Reading:

If you wish to delve into this topic for more detailed and specific information, try these resources.

http://www.webmd.com/ibs/

http://www.webmd.com/ibd-crohns-disease/

http://www.nlm.nih.gov/medlineplus/encyclopedia.html

http://www.mayoclinic.com/health-information/

https://www.verywell.com/ibs-4014702/

https://www.verywell.com/ibd-crohns-colitis-4014703

http://en.wikipedia.org/wiki/Dietary_fiber

http://umm.edu/health/medical/altmed/supplement/fiber

http://www.giforkids.com/

IBS for Dummies: available in e-book and print formats

Internet Resources

The following internet sites provide useful information. They were all active at time of publication.

CalorieCount.com Calorie and Nutrition Data
Searchable database providing nutritional information, including total fiber.
http://caloriecount.com/

CalorieKing Food Database
Searchable food directory that includes total fiber content and nutrient breakdown.
http://www.calorieking.com/foods/

WebMD Fiber-O-Meter
WebMD offers total fiber content and other nutritional information for more than 7000 foods via drill-down search.
http://www.webmd.com/diet/healthtool-fiber-meter

HighFiberDiet Fiber Lookup
Provides calories and total fiber for over 6000 foods via drill-down search.
http://www.highfiberdiet.net/

DietFacts Fast-Food Restaurant Nutrition Facts
Includes nutritional information (with total fiber content) for over 500 fast-food restaurants.
http://www.dietfacts.com/fastfood.asp

Bristol Stool Scale
Just what is normal stool, anyway?
http://en.wikipedia.org/wiki/Bristol_Stool_Scale
http://www.gutsense.org/constipation/normal_stools.html

Free Short Stories

I hope the following two stories will brighten your next few minutes, especially if you and the bathroom are bosom buddies right now.

How not to Prepare for a Colonoscopy

By D. Lee Jackson

"You haven't had one in over five years," my doctor said. "It's past time for another, especially since they removed polyps in your last one."

And with that, I was on my way to learning how *not* to prepare for a colonoscopy.

I'd had two previously, neither of which were fun. The reason? The purge required prior to each exam. A purge is exactly what it sounds like: a forced emptying of your entire colon so that the doctor can see inside you with a camera. To do it, you must take some sort of chemical concoction which induces your colon to empty itself in a shockingly abrupt manner over several hours.

I'd received different liquids for each of my previous exams. The first consisted of more than a gallon of some semi-lemonish slimy substance that made me vomit as well as purge, essentially cleaning out both ends. The second was a small green bottle of carbonated something which kept purging me until I thought it would take my liver with it.

Neither of those was as bad as this go-around.

I thought I would get lucky at first. My gastroenterologist gave me a dual-dose medicine, with instructions to take it at 5:00 and 9:00 the evening before the procedure. I mixed the first dose and downed it along with extra water, as indicated in the documentation. The oddly-sweet cocktail made me a little dizzy and a tad nauseous, but nothing as bad as what I'd experienced in the past. The purge actually progressed easily over the first couple of hours.

Then I read the purge medication's inactive ingredients.

Ingredients: *don't know that one, don't know that either, don't know ... wait. Sucralose. Uh-oh.*

I have a food allergy. To sucralose, an artificial sweetener. It gives me hives that usually show up a couple of weeks after I ingest it. One such outbreak covered half of my chest and stomach and lasted a week. And there it was, at the end of the list, buried deep within the patient information packet.

Damn.

I called the doctor's office and got his answering service. A doctor did return my call, but not the one who was going to perform the procedure. This doctor had no knowledge of my medical history, which includes a failed gastric bypass. Regardless, he told me to have my wife purchase a bottle of something called *magnesium citrate*, and said to take it instead for my second dose that evening.

If there was ever a substance that should be called *firewater*, magnesium citrate is it.

It didn't taste terrible at first. Sort of a hyper-fizzy lemony taste, although it did pucker my tongue. That was just the first few ounces, however. I had ten ounces of this devil's brew to finish.

By the time I made it halfway through the flask, I felt queasy. My bypass pouch wasn't happy with what I was forcing into it, so I slowed down my intake in response. When the queasiness faded, I'd resume drinking the liquid brimstone.

Lather. Rinse. Repeat.

Major problems set in as I consumed the last ounce. A burning sensation hit my stomach, mild at first, then progressively more intense. It spread to the center of my abdomen and eventually hit the level of *excruciating*. I felt like I'd been run through by a rod of white-hot steel. I couldn't move away from the kitchen sink. All I could do was lean on the counter and groan.

The nausea returned, so I tried to make it to our bathroom. I only managed five or six steps before calling for my wife's aid, something I've only done in the past when I've been sick enough to wind up in the hospital. This time, though, I just wanted her to help me make it to the bathroom. She did that, with me leaning on her back the entire way—a remarkable show of trust in my ability to keep her shirt clean, I must admit. Once we finally made it to the bathroom, she waited and watched while I positioned myself in front of the purge portal.

Now, please understand this: at 350 pounds, I am no featherweight. I also have arthritic knees and damaged kneecaps. This combination does not work well when applied to a ceramic tile floor. Hence, I grabbed a couple of folded bath towels, put them on the floor, and got down on both knees, waiting for the inevitable.

My memory from this point until about thirty minutes later is sketchy. I recall yelling, if not outright screaming, in frequent pain. My wife asked me at one point if I needed to go to a hospital. I also remember straightening out my toes so that my bare feet were parallel to the floor.

That last bit was a big mistake. More on it in a second.

After the proverbial *seemed like an eternity* period, my pain and nausea subsided enough for me realize that I had other things to deal with (i.e., the purge). I needed to switch ends on the toilet to avoid an impromptu wall paint job. I managed to get my right leg and foot into the proper position for standing, but my left knee couldn't handle the pressure despite the towel cushion. Once more, I called for my wife and asked her to help me up. Between her pulling me up and my pushing off the floor with my flattened left foot, I finally got upright, but not without letting out a true scream of sudden pain. I didn't know what I'd done, and frankly, I didn't care. At least I had the right end pointed the proper direction.

The purge continued to the point where I was letting out what felt like pure battery acid. I'm surprised it didn't etch the porcelain of the toilet, considering what it was doing to the rest of my body. Thankfully, the whole ordeal began to let up at about 11:30 p.m., after more than two hours of firewater-induced hell.

And for some reason, my left foot hurt.

The remainder of the preparation and the exam itself were, surprisingly, rather easy on me. However, my foot continued to hurt—specifically, the number two toe on my left foot. The doctors in the procedure room examined it (I'm guessing most of the feet they've seen have been up people's rears) and said I'd broken it, damaged the joint, or injured a ligament when my wife helped me stand. In any case, there was nothing that could be done for it other than to *buddy tape* it to the adjacent toe for support and keep it elevated.

Believe it or not, I have two positives that I can take with me from the whole experience. First, I had no polyps. Second, due to the inordinate length and twisting of my colon, I might get to have a CT scan colonoscopy next time around instead of having a doctor put another camera up my rear. As long as it doesn't involve sucralose, firewater, broken toes, or battery acid bowel movements, I might actually consent to the procedure.

Broccoli Blues

By Kathy Steinemann

This is a piece from *Nag Nag Nag: Megan and Emmett Volume I*, a family humor anthology published in 2015.

If you're allergic to laughter, get your meds ready. *Nag Nag Nag* will exercise your laugh muscles. It might even make you wet your pants.

Megan and Emmett share many of the same quirks and problems as other married couples. The way they deal with them might take you aback.

Discover how Emmett copes with Megan's nagging. Learn how Megan treats telemarketers. Her once-in-a-lifetime offer makes them hang up. Every time. Will Emmett ever fix the blasted dishwasher? You'll be shocked when you realize why it broke in the first place. And how does he get around Megan's cat rules?

Granddaughters, Violet and Lisa, provide a few surprises and chuckles too, with the unique perspectives of youth. Their widowed mother, Marsha, is determined to raise her daughters right. That means healthy food like broccoli. Yuck! The difference between broccoli and snot is that kids don't eat broccoli.

And we can't forget Sabrina, the Siamese cat. You'll find her meowing and purring her way into your heart as she careens around corners and wins the affections of the most unlikely characters.

Nag Nag Nag will entertain you with laughs, tears, and unexpected twists.

Lisa is sick, and she's sure the broccoli caused it.

~*~

Marsha felt Lisa's forehead and took the thermometer from her mouth. "No temperature. Still have tummy cramps?"

Lisa grimaced. "Uh huh. I'm sorry I pooped my pants. I runned to the bathroom fast as I could, but my runs runned faster than me."

Marsha stroked her daughter's hair. "I don't think it's serious, but I'll see if I can make a doctor's appointment for you."

A giant rumbling noise exploded from under the covers. Lisa frowned. "It's okay. I just farted."

Her mother tsk-tsked. "What do you say?"

"Thank-you?"

"You excuse yourself when you fart."

"Oh. I forgot. 'Xcuse me. It's broccoli that made me sick. Grampa says the only difference between broccoli and snot is kids don't eat broccoli. And I hate it. It was yucky broccoli … broccoli … broccoli."

"Nice try. Broccoli is *healthy*, and I haven't served it for over a week. You had oatmeal for breakfast. That shouldn't make you sick. Next time I make broccoli, I'll smother it with a cheesy sauce."

Lisa threw off the covers and dashed for the bathroom.

Marsha followed her and waited by the open door. "Don't use so much toilet paper. You only have a tiny butt."

"Then you should use a *whole bunch* for *your* butt, Mommy."

Marsha sighed. Maybe it was time to stop finishing off the girls' leftovers. "You okay?"

"Yup. Now my tummy doesn't hurt."

Marsha grabbed the phone, had a lengthy discussion with the nurse, and scheduled a doctor's appointment for 3 p.m.

She considered cancelling after Lisa's dramatic improvement throughout the morning, but decided to be safe.

~*~

They arrived fifteen minutes early.

The waiting room overflowed with mothers and kids. A single father entertained his daughter. Occasionally his gaze wandered around the room. He reminded Marsha of a guy in the bar checking out the female customers. Not that she'd been to a bar recently. The man's eyes rested on her ring finger for a fleeting moment, spotted her wedding band, and flitted away.

Marsha slumped in her seat. It had been over five years since she'd lost Paul in a motorcycle accident while she was pregnant with Lisa, their second child. Some days she was so lonely. ... But she wasn't ready to move on.

A little boy in the chair next to Lisa wiggled closer. "Are you sick?"

Lisa leaned away from him. "You're not s'pposed to get near people in the doctor's office. You might get Germans."

He giggled. "Germs, stoopid. 'Sides, I'm not sick. I got a itchy ... you know." He rubbed at his crotch.

Lisa wrinkled her nose and stared at the boy's fingers. "Maybe you got germ-meezles on your weenie."

His mother cleared her throat and frowned at both kids. The boy bit his lip, continuing to scratch as he returned his attention to his handheld video game.

After a lengthy wait, the nurse summoned Marsha and Lisa to an examination room.

She closed the door and turned to Lisa. "I'm Faye. Your mommy told me all about your problems when I talked to her on the phone. She wants us to give you a complete checkup. Before Dr. Eunice gets here, I'll do a couple of things to make her job easier, okay?"

Lisa clung to Marsha's side for a moment before nodding.

Faye took Lisa's temperature and then patted the little girl's shoulder with gloved fingertips. "Can you stand on one foot?"

Lisa cocked her head. Lines formed on her brow. She stepped forward and stood on one of the nurse's feet.

Faye giggled. "That's not what I meant, sweetie. Can you stand like a ballet dancer, with one foot in the air and the other on the floor?"

Lisa pirouetted and stopped, arms outstretched, while she balanced on one foot.

"Good. Your balance seems fine. Now we'll check your hydration and sugar levels. I'm going to give you this plastic cup, and I'd like you to pee into it. The bathroom is down the hall to your right. Afterward, Mommy can bring you back here, and Dr. Eunice will be able to see you soon."

Lisa wrinkled her nose as she stared into the cup. "Do I hafta drink it?"

Faye snorted. "Nope. We put a little stick of cardboard in your pee and wait for it to turn color."

Lisa's eyes widened. "Is it magic cardboard?"

"Yup."

She smiled. "My Grampa is magic, but he doesn't have cardboard that changes color."

~*~

Bathroom duties complete, Marsha and Lisa waited for the doctor's knock. Dr. Eunice stepped into the room.

Lisa beamed. She could see a lump in the doctor's lab jacket. Candy. Dr. E. gave away the tastiest candies. Ever.

The doctor reviewed Lisa's chart. "So, diarrhea, gas, and tummy cramps, but no fever."

Lisa shook her head. "Direeeeeeeea!"

Mother and doctor shared an amused glance.

Dr. Eunice snickered as she typed a few characters on her laptop. "Has this happened before?"

Marsha shrugged. "A few times, but not this severe."

"Can you recall what Lisa ate each time she had these symptoms?"

"Oatmeal today ... chocolate milkshake a couple of days ago ... cornflakes over the weekend ... ice cream cone last week. Something different each time."

Dr. Eunice's eyes crinkled. "Different, but not so different. All the foods you mentioned have something in common: dairy."

Marsha slapped her forehead. "Of course. I should have thought of that. Dad has lactose intolerance. Is there a test you can do to confirm it?"

Lisa squirmed. "I don't want any tests. Violet says they're horrrror-bull. You gotta study for them. And 'sides, I'm not in school yet."

The doctor grinned. "Not that kind of test. But no need to worry. We don't do lactose intolerance tests for kids. Just stay away from dairy or eat lactose-free products."

"I always stay away from Barry. He's mean."

Dr. Eunice handed Lisa a candy in a gleaming gold wrapper. "That's good. You stay away from Barry and milk and cheese and ice cream. I'll give your mommy a pamphlet that explains all about your tummy problem. Remember to take your vitamins and eat healthy."

"You mean I still hafta eat broccoli? And I can't have ice cream?" Her face wrinkled as though she had just sucked on a lemon.

"If you have a little bit of ice cream, it will give you gas, and you shouldn't get a tummy ache. But *only* a little bit. Okay?"

Lisa beamed. "Yeah. Then I can ask Grampa to pull on *my* finger from now on."

Books by Kathy Steinemann

Humor
• Nag Nag Nag: Megan and Emmett Volume I

Speculative Fiction
• Envision: Future Fiction

Multiple Genre
• Suppose: Drabbles, Flash Fiction, and Short Stories

Alternate History
• Vanguard of Hope: Sapphire Brigade Book 1
• The Doctor's Deceit: Sapphire Brigade Book 2

Nonfiction
• CreateSpace Graphics Primer
• IBS-IBD Fiber Charts
• The IBS Compass
• Practical and Effective Tips for Learning Foreign Languages
• Top Tips for Packing Your Suitcase
• Top Tips for Travel by Air

Multilingual
• Life, Death and Consequences
• Leben, Tod und Konsequenzen (German Edition)
• Matthew and the Pesky Ants
• Matthias und die verflixten Ameisen (German Edition)

About the Author

Kathy Steinemann, Grandma Birdie to her grandkids, lives in the foothills on the Alberta side of the Canadian Rocky Mountains. She has loved writing for as long as she can remember.

As a young child, she scribbled poems and stories. During the progression of her love affair with words, she won public-speaking and writing awards, and she contributed to her school newspaper. Then every Monday, rain or shine, she walked home instead of taking the bus so that she could deliver her latest column to the community weekly.

Her career has taken varying directions, including positions as editor of a small-town paper, computer-network administrator, and webmaster. She has also worked on projects in commercial art and cartooning.

Kathy has suffered from IBS for several years. During a particularly intense and extended attack that lasted for months, she tried to locate as many details as possible about this often-debilitating condition. It was difficult to obtain data for soluble fiber.

She decided to write this book, and always carries a copy with her to restaurants and grocery stores.

Kathy's Website

KathySteinemann.com

Afterword

I'd like to talk to you now about reviews.

Positive comments and ratings help authors earn a living. Please take a few moments to post an online review.

Your feedback and support are greatly appreciated.

You have reached the end of the book. Thank you for reading. If you enjoyed it, please recommend it to a friend.

If you're reading this book and did not pay for it, or it was not purchased for your use only, please buy your own copy.

Made in the USA
San Bernardino, CA
15 October 2016